# SYNTHETIC ORGANS

## and Other Medical Tech

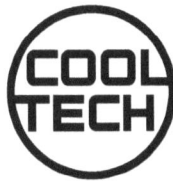

Co-published by agreement between Shi Tu Hui and World Book, Inc.

Shi Tu Hui
Room 1807, Block 1,
#3 West Dawang Road
Chaoyang District, Beijing 100025
P.R. China

World Book, Inc
180 North LaSalle Street
Suite 900
Chicago, Illinois 60601
USA

Library of Congress Cataloging-in-Publication Data for this volume has been applied for.

Cool Tech (set #2)
ISBN: 978-0-7166-5387-5 (set, hc)

Synthetic Organs and Other Medical Tech
ISBN: 978-0-7166-5393-6 (hc)

Also available as:
ISBN: 978-0-7166-5399-8 (e-book)
ISBN: 978-0-7166-5405-6 (soft cover)

Written by Alex Woolf

## STAFF

VP, Editorial: Tom Evans

Manager, New Product: Nicholas Kilzer

Curriculum Designer: Caroline Davidson

Proofreader: Nathalie Strassheim

Coordinator, Design Development & Production:
  Brenda Tropinski

Senior Media Editor: Rosalia Bledsoe

Developed with World Book by
White-Thomson Publishing LTD

www.wtpub.co.uk

# ACKNOWLEDGMENTS

COVER  © Mauro Fermariello, Science Photo Library
5-7  © Shutterstock
8-9  © Ella Maru Studio/Science Photo Library; © Adrian Mars, Shutterstock; © Satnam Singh, Deepak Choudhury, Fang Yu, Vladimir Mironov, May Win Naing; © Miriam Doerr & Martin Frommherz, Shutterstock
10-11  © James King-Holmes, Science Photo Library; © Elena Pavlovich, Shutterstock; HIA (licensed under CC BY-SA 3.0); © Noctiluxx/iStock
12-13  © imtmphoto/Shutterstock; © Yuuji/iStock
14-15  © kanetmark/Shutterstock; © Canan Dagdeviren; © Harvard Medical School; © Orawan Pattarawimonchai, Shutterstock; © HASPhotos/Shutterstock; © Nicola_K_ photos/Shutterstock
16-21  © Shutterstock
22-23  © Love Employee/Shutterstock; © Ira Dvilyuk, Shutterstock; © goffkein.pro/Shutterstock; © Laguna Design/Science Photo Library; © Alexander Raths, Shutterstock
24-25  © metamorworks/Shutterstock; © Hryshchyshen Serhii, Shutterstock
26-29  © Shutterstock
30-31  © Gorodenkoff/Shutterstock; © Science Photo Library/

Alamy Images; © aastock/Shutterstock; © Nuk2013/ Shutterstock
32-33  © Monopoly919/Shutterstock; © Gorodenkoff/ Shutterstock
34-35  © Peter Menzel, Science Photo Library; © Phanie/Alamy Images; © MAD.vertise/Shutterstock; © MedicalWorks/ Shutterstock
36-37  © Sipa USA/Alamy Images; © Jbruiz/Shutterstock; © Zapp2Photo/Shutterstock; © Roomie
38-39  © Vereshchagin Dmitry, Shutterstock; © Ehrlich Michael, Zaidel Yuval, Weiss Patrice L., Melamed Yekel Arie, Gefen Naomi, Supic Lazar, Ezra Tsur Elishai; © Miriam Doerr & Martin Frommherz, Shutterstock; © Philippe Psaila, Science Photo Library
40-41  © Anton Gvozdikov, Shutterstock; © Frame Stock Footage/Shutterstock
42-43  © Jens Meyer, AP Photo; © MangKangMangMee/ Shutterstock; © Patrick Landmann, Science Photo Library; © Fit Ztudio/Shutterstock
44-45  © Newman Studio/Shutterstock; © Ground Picture/ Shutterstock; J.M. Eddins Jr., U.S. Air Force; © Thierry Berrod, Mona Lisa Production/Science Photo Library

# CONTENTS

There is a glossary of terms on the first page. Terms defined in the glossary are in boldface type that **looks like this** on their first appearance on any spread (two facing pages).

# GLOSSARY

**algorithm** a set of step-by-step instructions written in code that a computer can use to perform a task.

**app** short for software application. A software application is a computer program that enables a human user to perform some task or activity.

**autonomous** able to operate with little or no human control or intervention.

**chatbot** a computer program designed to simulate conversation with human users, especially over the internet.

**console** a computer terminal where a user may input commands and view output.

**5G** refers to the 5th generation cellular network—the most advanced global wireless technology designed to connect nearly everyone and everything through smartphones, computers, and other devices.

**fluorescent** any substance that glows when exposed to certain kinds of energy.

**haptic** technology that can create an experience of touch through forces, vibrations, or motions to a user.

**laser** a device that produces a powerful beam of light. Such a beam can travel over long distances or be tightly focused to a small diameter.

**microprocessor** the central unit of a computer system that performs arithmetic and logic operations.

**orthopedic** a branch of medicine that focuses on the care of the musculoskeletal system. This system consists of muscles, bones, joints, ligaments, and tendons.

**pandemic** a widespread occurrence of an infectious disease over a whole country or the world at a particular time.

**prosthetic** a device designed to replace a missing part of the body or to make a part of the body work better.

**protein** a substance made up of amino acids. Proteins are complex organic compounds that are essential to the functioning as well as the structure of all organic cells.

**rehabilitate** restore someone to health or normal life by training and therapy following illness or injury.

**skin graft** a surgical operation in which a piece of healthy skin is transplanted to a new site on the body.

**symptoms** any feeling of illness or physical or mental change that is caused by a disease. Muscle aches and fever are symptoms of the flu.

**synthetic** an artificial substance or material.

**transplant** to surgically transfer an organ or tissue from one part or individual to another.

# INTRODUCTION

Imagine a world where hearts can be printed, and tiny machines in our bodies constantly monitor our health. We can obtain round-the-clock medical advice from an intelligent virtual assistant. And if we need to visit a hospital, we are cared for and even operated on by robots. Such a world may sound fanciful, but these technologies are already in development and may appear sooner than you think.

When our organs fail, doctors may need to replace them. Today, replacement organs only come from human donors. But that is all set to change. Soon, thanks to bioprinting and stem cell technology, organs, tissues, bones, and blood vessels will be made to order in a laboratory.

Advances in computer technology are making medical care increasingly personalized and data-driven. Wearable devices and implants will allow us to take control of our health. These medical devices will alert us to any problems at an early stage, leading to prompt treatment and faster recovery.

Artificial intelligence (AI) today plays an ever greater role in the diagnosis and treatment of disease. Robots will provide care and companionship for people living with long-term medical conditions. Virtual reality (VR) will help patients deal with physical and mental pain. In the more distant future, miniature nanorobots may work inside us, destroying viruses and cancer cells as they emerge. This book looks at the many ways in which medical tech is going to transform health care provision in the coming decades.

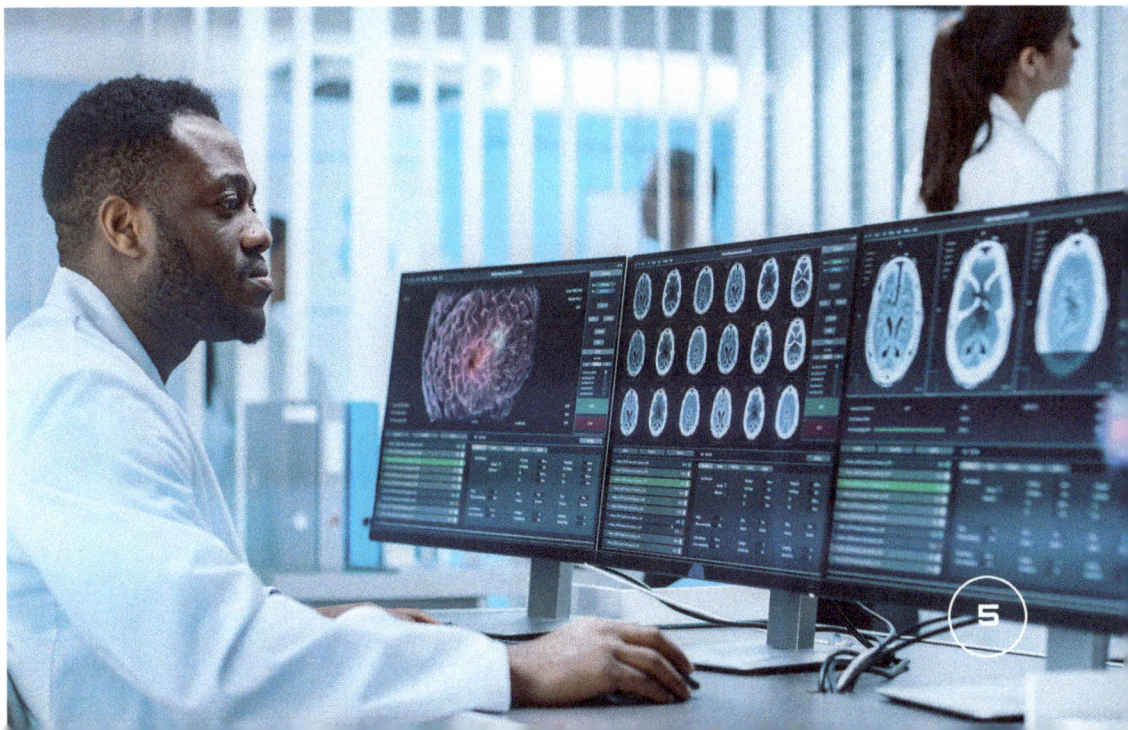

# 1 SYNTHETIC ORGANS

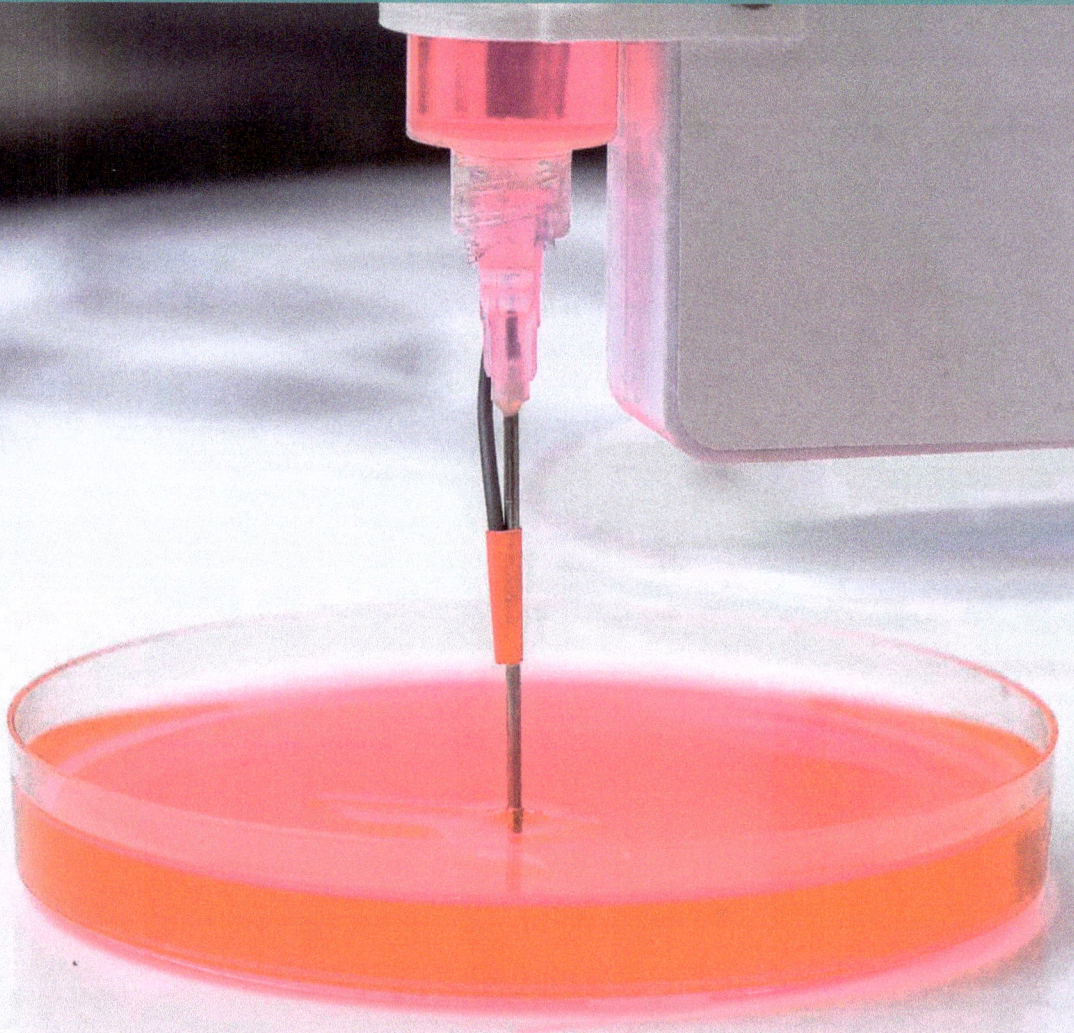

# ENDING OUR RELIANCE ON HUMAN DONORS

The human body is a complex machine. Each organ plays its part in keeping us alive and healthy. Sadly, our organs occasionally fail and must be repaired or replaced. Many people kindly choose to donate their healthy organs for use after their death. However, there is a global shortage of donor organs. Around the world, critically ill people wait for donor kidneys, hearts, livers, and lungs. Now, technology offers a solution: organs custom-created in a laboratory. **Synthetic** organs can be grown from human stem cells, or they can be 3D-printed—a process known as bioprinting.

These technologies offer an important advantage beyond a potentially limitless supply of donor organs—compatibility. A patient's immune system often rejects organs donated by another. **Transplant** patients who have received a new organ must take medicines to suppress their immune systems to prevent rejection. But this leaves them vulnerable to infection. Synthetic organs use cells from the patient's own body, thereby lowering the risk of rejection.

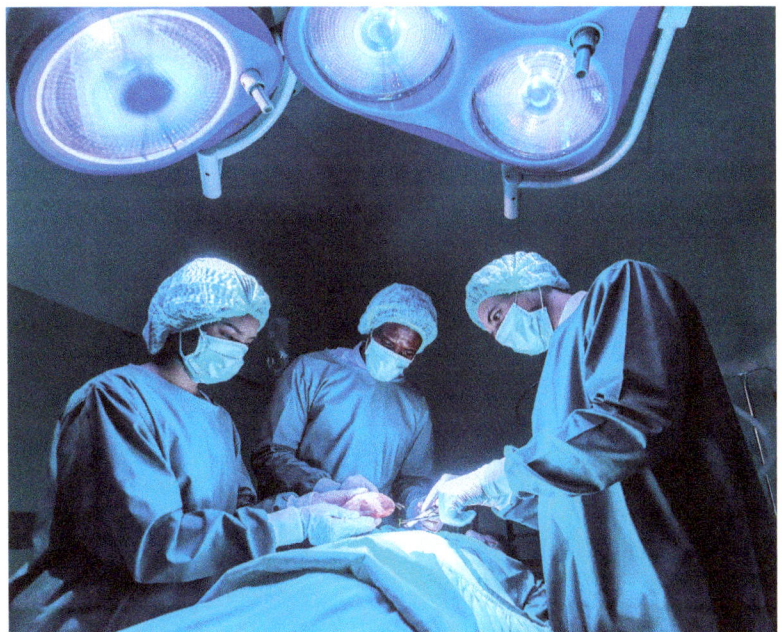

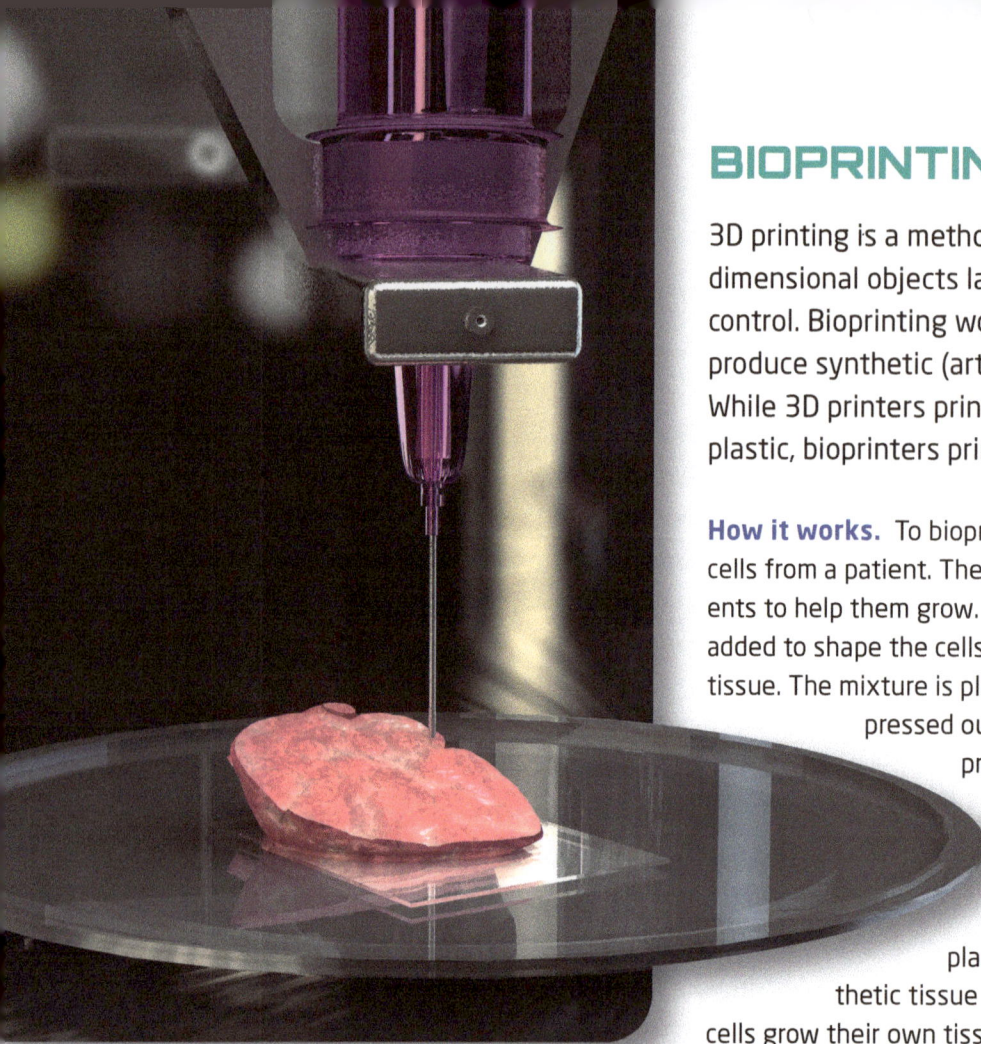

# BIOPRINTING

3D printing is a method of constructing three-dimensional objects layer by layer under computer control. Bioprinting works in a similar way to produce synthetic (artificial) human body parts. While 3D printers print with liquid or powdered plastic, bioprinters print with living cells!

**How it works.** To bioprint an organ, doctors take cells from a patient. They feed the cells with nutrients to help them grow. A special gel called bioink is added to shape the cells into a structure like living tissue. The mixture is placed in the bioprinter and pressed out one layer at a time. The printer is programmed to build the organ according to exact requirements based on data from patient scans. Once the organ is placed inside the body, the synthetic tissue breaks down and the organ's cells grow their own tissue to replace it.

**Progress.** Organs are complex structures with different tissues fed by networks of blood vessels. Researchers are not yet able to bioprint a functioning human organ. But they have made progress on simpler body parts. In 2017, Australian surgeons fitted a bioprinted shinbone into a patient's leg. In 2018, a British lab printed the first human corneas. In 2019, American scientists developed a method of printing living skin and blood vessels. These could provide **skin grafts** for burn victims. In 2022, an American woman received a bioprinted ear.

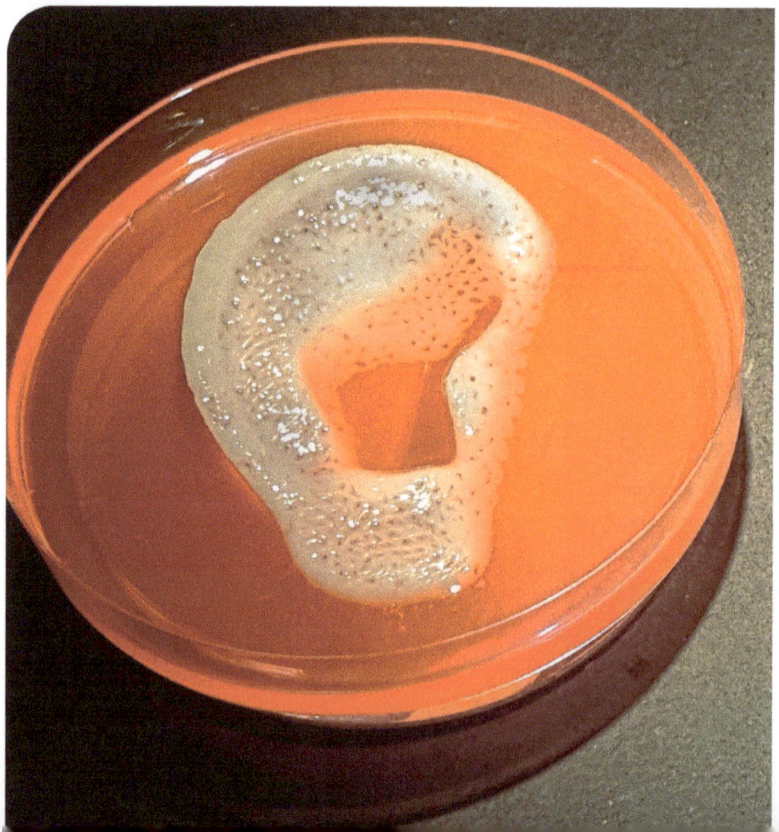

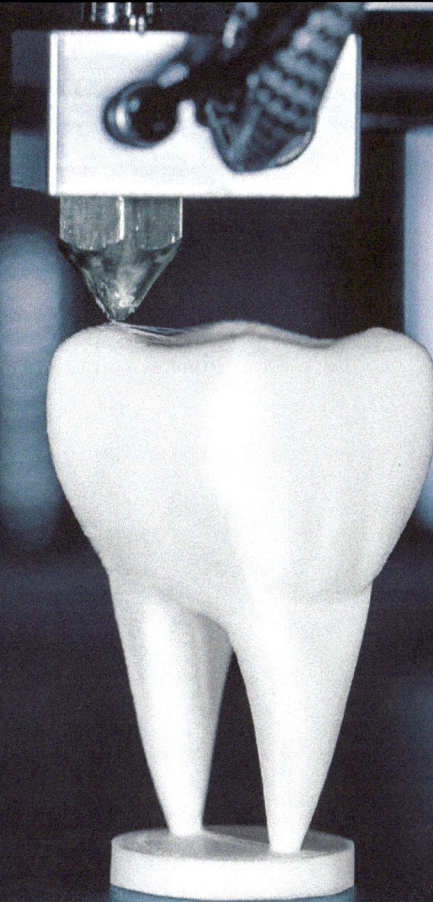

**Prosthetics and implants.** When patients simply require a replacement part, the process is much easier. Traditional 3D printing can create hip and knee replacements, dental implants, and **prosthetic** limbs from strong new materials. In 2021, a British man was fitted with a 3D-printed false eye. 3D-printed prosthetics and implants are relatively cheap to make and can be perfectly fitted to the patient.

**In situ bioprinting.** Researchers are working on technology that will allow living cells, bones, and even organs to be printed within the body during surgery. This technology will make surgery less invasive and improve patient recovery time. However, developing a fast-setting bioink remains a challenge.

3D printing is already proving useful in a variety of applications and industries. The printers can produce objects small or large to meet almost any design and engineering need. Some 3D-printed objects may even be used in the human body!

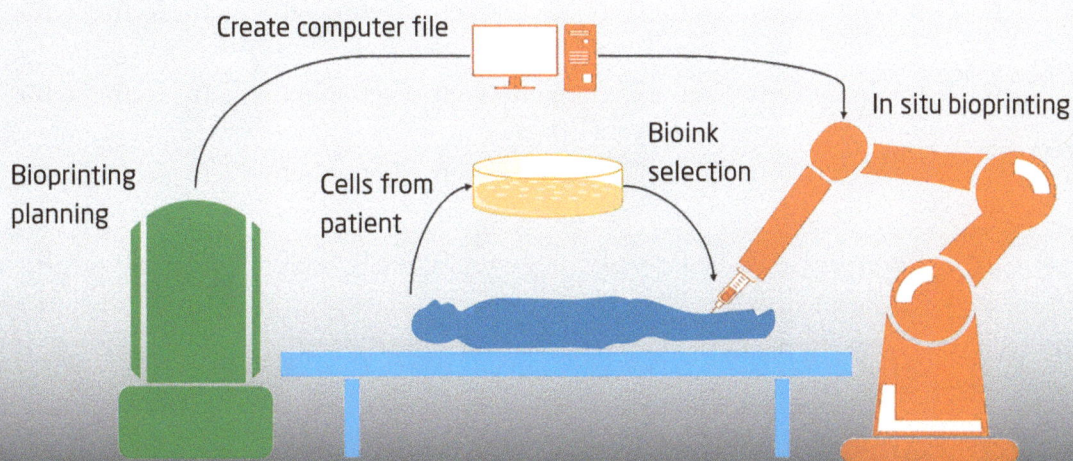

Create computer file

Bioink selection

In situ bioprinting

Bioprinting planning

Cells from patient

# TISSUE ENGINEERING

Our body tissues are composed of cells that grow within a scaffold that gives them shape. Each organ has its own specialized cells. Tissue engineering uses the body's own cells combined with synthetic or natural scaffolds to repair or build new tissue.

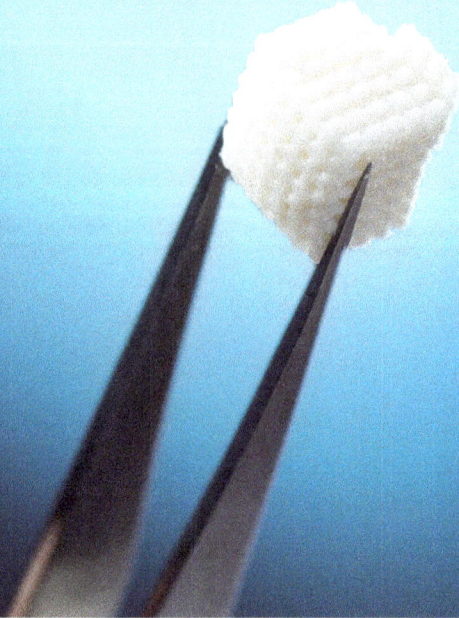

**Building the scaffold.** A scaffold provides a shape and structure for cells to grow new tissue. The natural scaffolds of our tissues are made of a **protein** called *collagen.* Scientists can build synthetic scaffolds from a wide range of materials, including proteins and plastics. This approach works for such simple body parts as the trachea (windpipe). For more complex structures, such as a heart, liver, lung, or kidney, scientists use the natural collagen scaffold and blood vessels of a donor organ with the original cells stripped away.

**Introducing new cells.** Once scientists create the scaffold, they introduce cells taken from the patient. They introduce *stem cells*—cells capable of generating any specialized cells for the organ to be rebuilt. Scientists usually add growth factors—substances that stimulate the stem cells to grow.

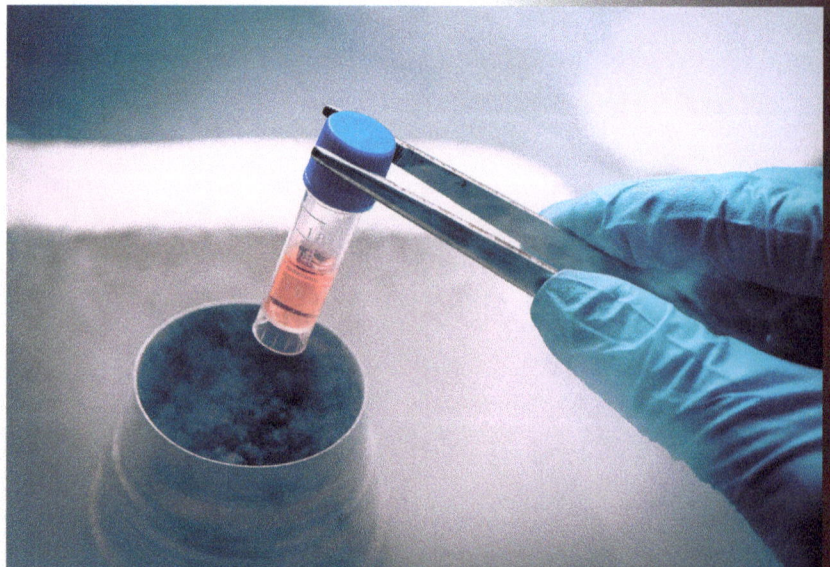

**Today.** Tissue engineering is currently in its infancy. Procedures are costly and experimental. Nevertheless, scientists have already built simple body parts and implanted them in patients. These structures include bladders, arteries, skin, cartilage, and even a windpipe. More complex organ tissues for the heart, lung, and liver have been successfully engineered in the lab. These are not yet ready to be implanted in patients. But they are used for research and for testing new medicines.

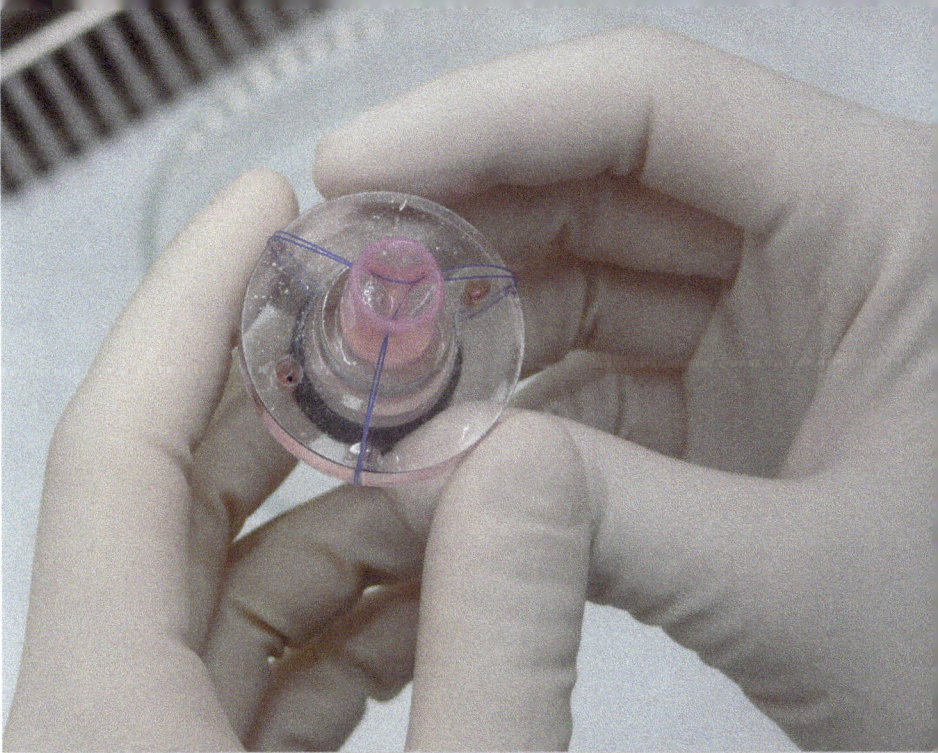

**Tomorrow.** The ultimate goal of tissue engineering is to engineer organs for transplantation. The kidney, heart, and lungs have an intricate architecture and a network of blood vessels. Once grown, synthetic organs must be kept alive for transplantation. Engineered muscle needs to be stretched. Engineered lungs need a regular flow of air. These are some of the challenges tissue engineers must overcome.

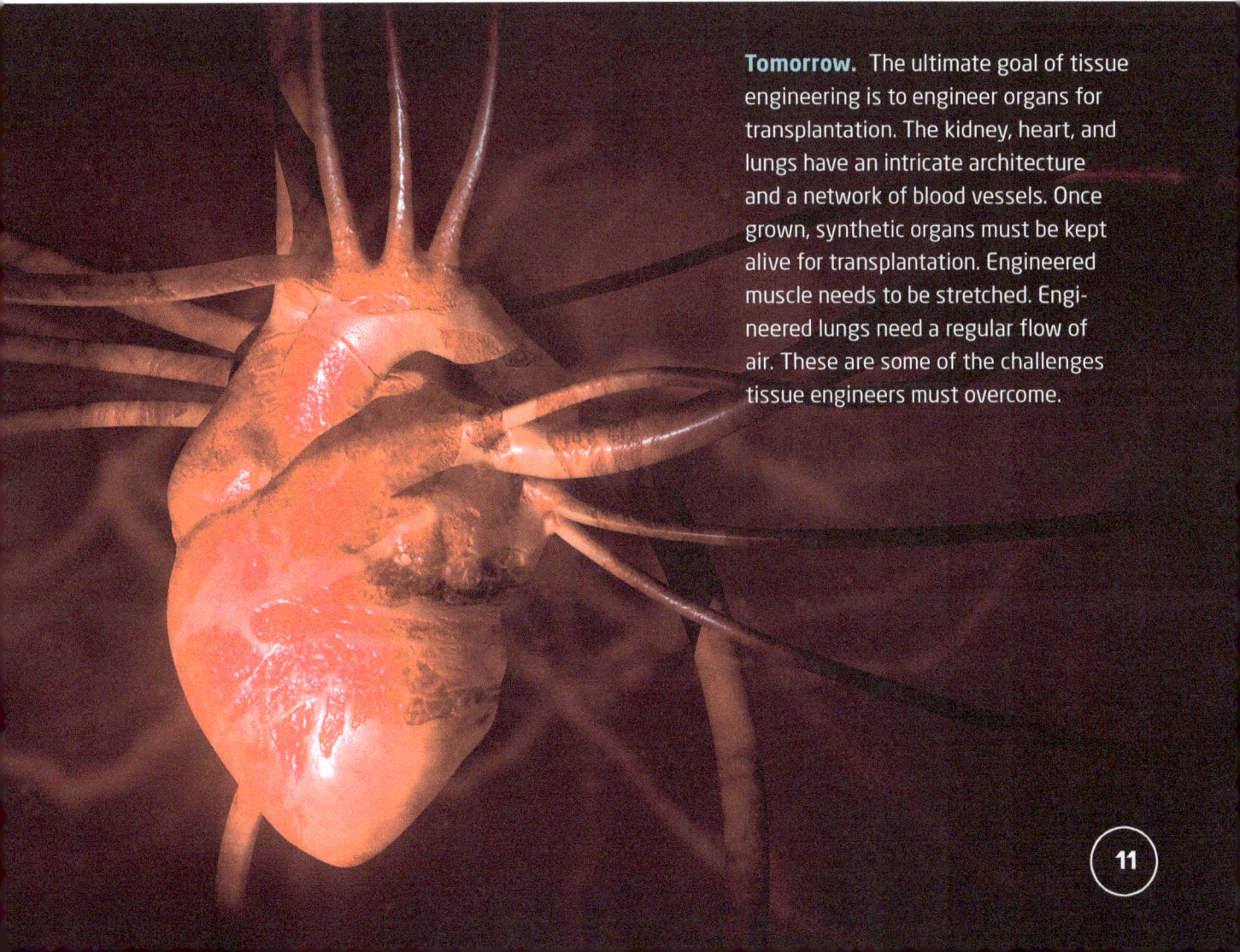

# 2 REMOTE MONITORING

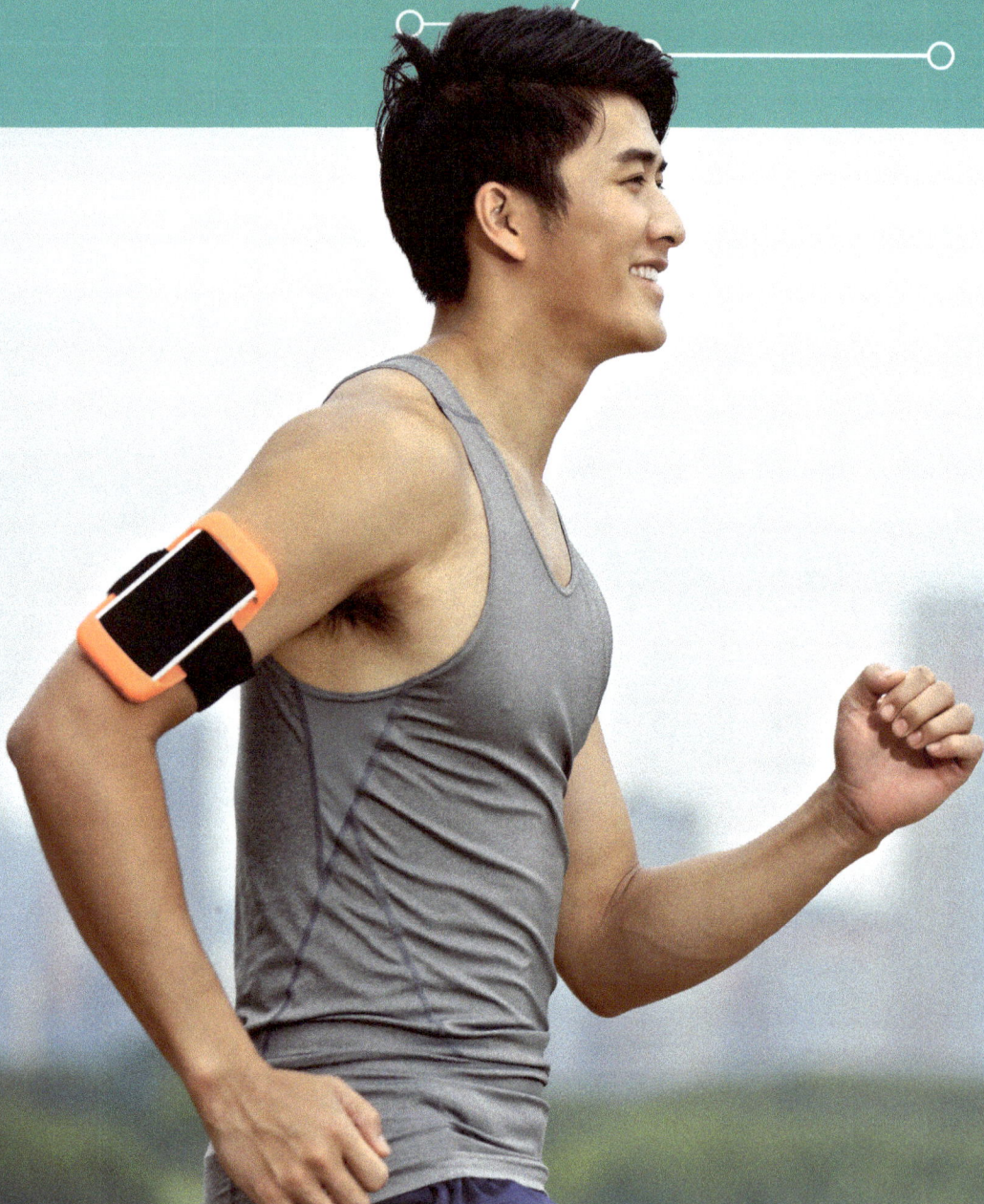

# TRACKING OUR HEALTH

Your body lets you know when something is wrong. You may feel pain or discomfort. But some ailments have no obvious **symptoms.** High blood pressure, high cholesterol, diabetes, sleep apnea (pauses in breathing while asleep), and some cancers rarely have obvious symptoms. Luckily, technology can help.

Today, patients can be alerted to medical problems as soon as they arise, thanks to an array of advanced health-tracking technologies. These include wearables—electronic devices worn as accessories, sewn into clothing, or even tattooed on skin. Wearables constantly check vital signs, such as our heart rate and blood pressure.

Electronic monitoring devices can also be implanted within the body. New "smart" implants give doctors real-time data on what is happening inside a patient. They may function as an early-warning system for disease.

Future health-monitoring devices will be connected to form a network known as the Internet of Medical Things (IoMT). The IoMT will give doctors a complete and up-to-date overview of a patient's health. This will be especially helpful for patients with long-term health care needs or those living in remote areas.

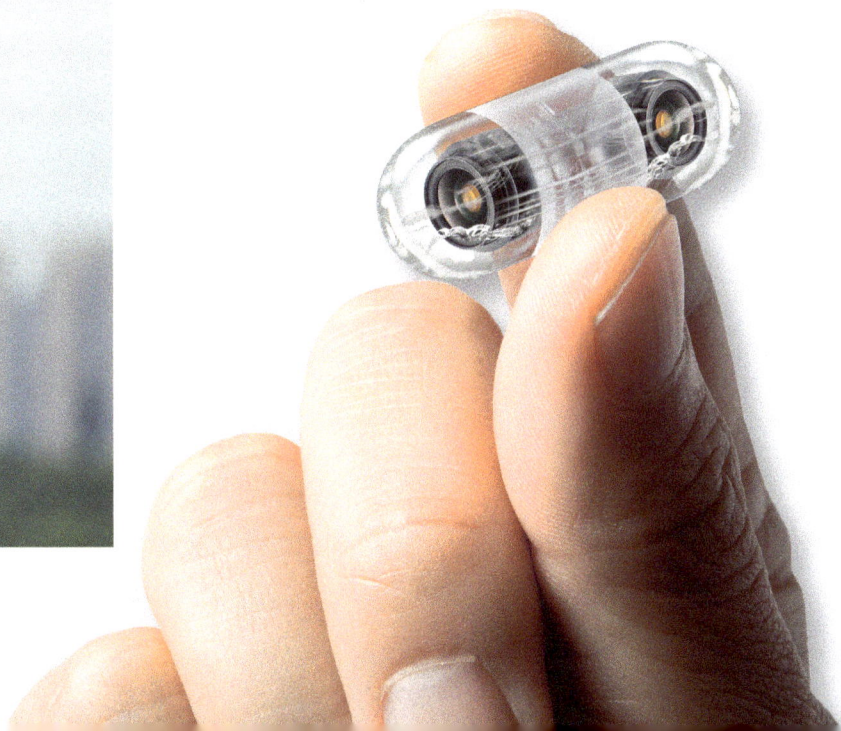

# WEARABLES

Medical wearables capture real-time data about a user's health and fitness. Wearable smartwatches, pedometers, activity trackers, or smart rings track steps, heart rate, and sleep patterns. New wearable tech can measure blood pressure and record electrical signals from the heart. They can warn patients of such emerging conditions as diabetes and irregular heartbeat.

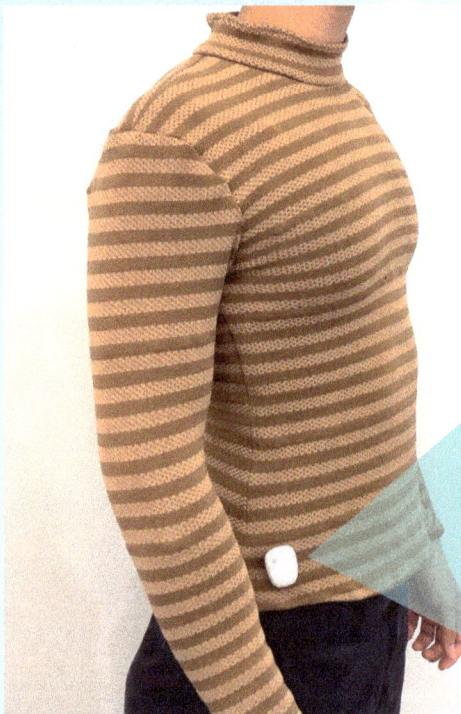

**Smart clothes.** Scientists are developing a small, lightweight sensor that can be sewn into a sweater to record the user's vital signs. The machine-washable sensor can be removed and placed in another garment. The **5G**-enabled sensor communicates with a patient's smartphone via an **app.** Other researchers are developing a smart shirt that can monitor lung health. The shirt is embedded with sensors that can diagnose asthma, pneumonia, bronchitis, and chronic obstructive pulmonary disease (COPD). The shirt sends the information to your smartphone.

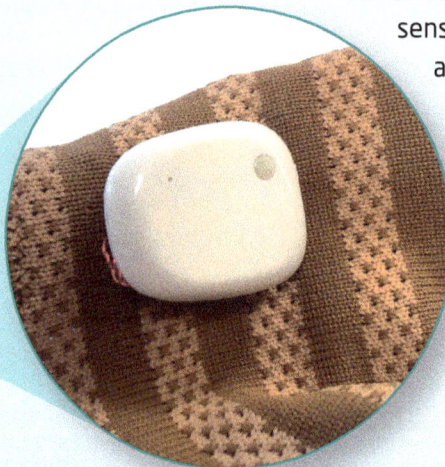

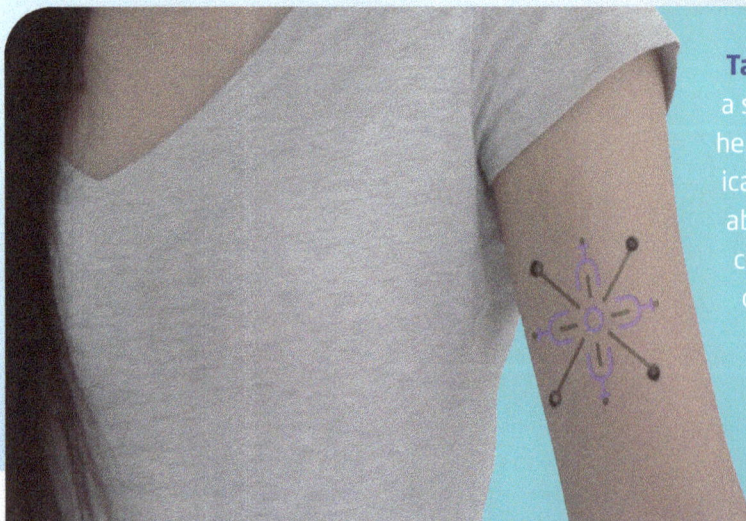

**Tattoos.** Researchers have developed a smart tattoo that can track your health. The tattoo ink reacts to chemicals in the skin to gain information about the wearer's blood. The tattoo changes color if you are dehydrated or alerts people with diabetes when their blood sugar levels rise. The tattoo also links to a smartphone app. Scientists plan to make the tattoo last only as long as it is needed.

**Smart hearing aids.** The latest hearing aids incorporate advanced health-tracking technology. They can track movement and heart rate and record body temperature (the ear is the best place to take this measurement). The hearing aids can also tell if the wearer has fallen and contact a caregiver or emergency medical services (EMS).

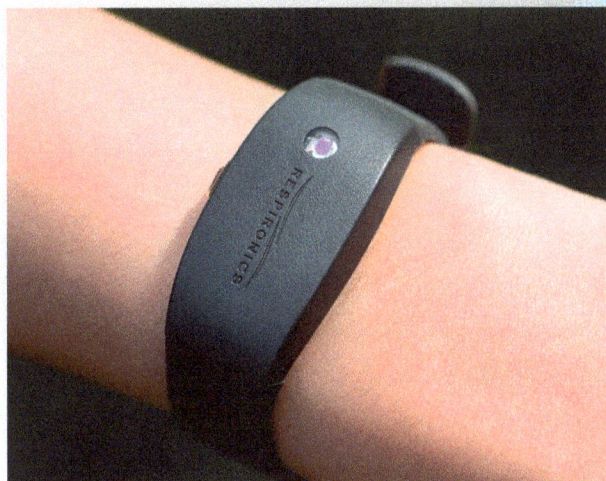

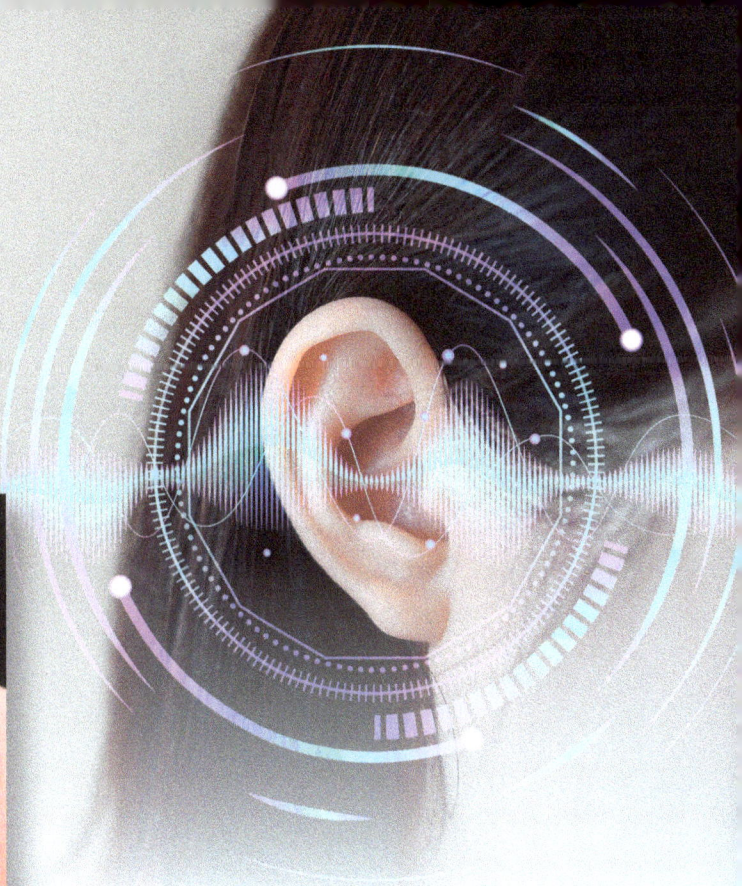

**Home health tracking.** Many patients suffering from *chronic* (long-term) illnesses, especially those living in remote areas, are using technology to monitor their health at home. The KardiaMobile heart monitor is a portable device for checking heart rhythm and electrical activity. The device is easy to use, and data is securely sent to the doctor via a smartphone app.

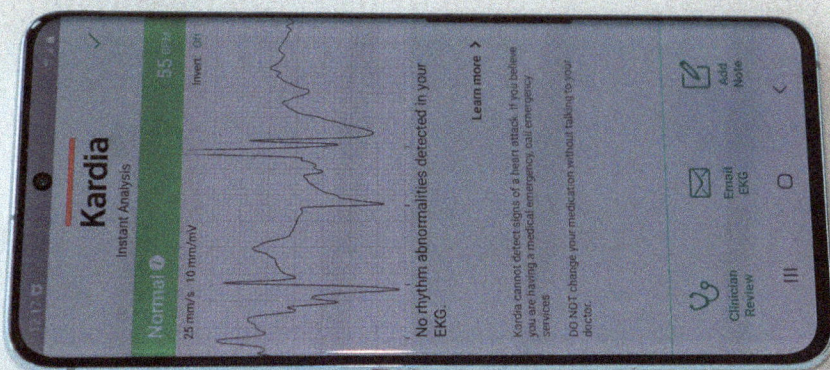

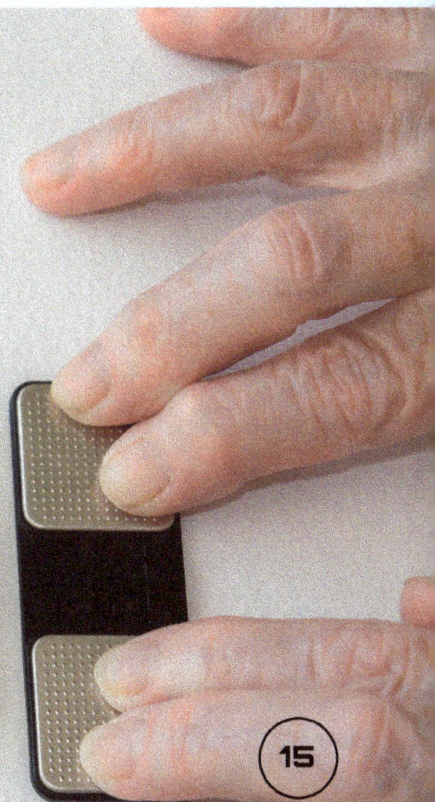

# SMART IMPLANTS

Some health information can only be obtained from devices implanted *within* the body. Wearables cannot do that. Smart implants equipped with sensors and **microprocessors** work inside the body to diagnose diseases, monitor a patient's condition, and even deliver treatments.

**Smart pills** are capsules swallowed by a patient that contain a camera and chemical sensors. The capsule records images and takes readings as it passes through the digestive system. The capsule may measure glucose levels, acidity, and core body temperature. It can also verify that a patient has taken medicine as directed and if it is effective. The data is wirelessly sent to a doctor. The latest smart pills contain sensors that locate the ideal environment and release medication. Future smart pills will analyze oxygen and carbon dioxide levels in the intestines—important markers of gut health.

**Stents.** A stent is a tiny tube of flexible material placed inside a narrowing blood vessel to open it up for better blood flow. Researchers have developed an electronic stent that can wirelessly transmit useful data such as blood pressure and pulse.

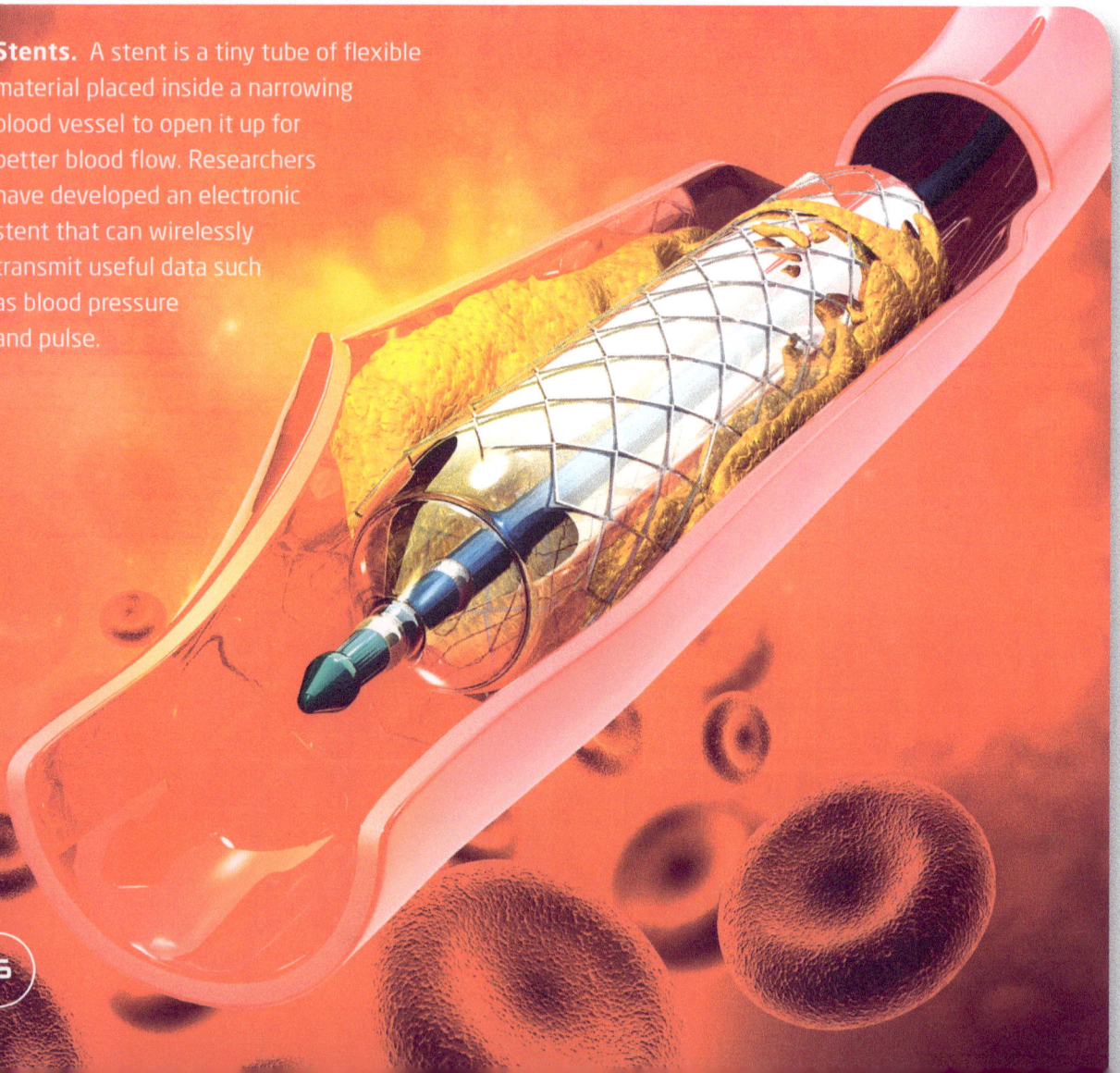

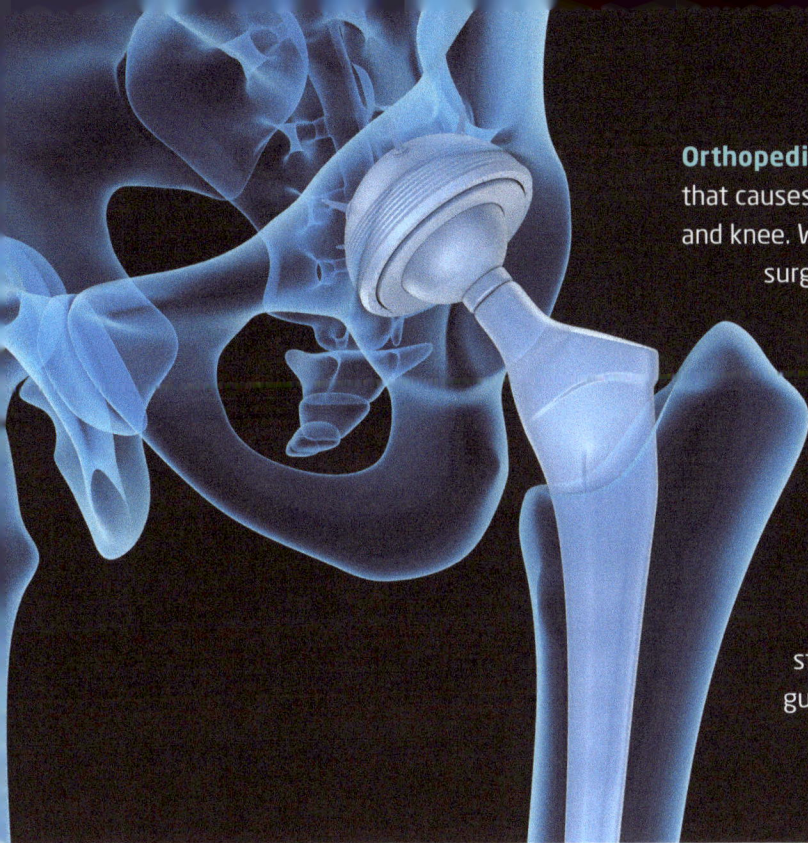

**Orthopedic implants.** Osteoarthritis is a disease that causes pain in the joints, especially the hip and knee. When serious, patients may undergo surgery for hip or knee replacement. This involves replacing the joint with an **orthopedic** implant to relieve pain and improve function. The latest implants are equipped with sensors and microprocessors to monitor a patient's condition after surgery. Sensors detect any loosening or failure of the implant, a patient's range of motion, stride length, gait, and muscle strength. Doctors use the information to guide a patient's treatment plan.

**Cardiac monitor.** Some heart conditions require long-term monitoring. An implantable loop cardiac monitor is a small (about the size of a paper clip) device inserted under the skin of the chest. It records the heart's electrical activity and alerts a patient or doctor of any abnormal heart rhythms. The latest monitors are equipped with a self-learning AI (artificial intelligence) **algorithm** that quickly adapts to a patient's heart to avoid false alarms.

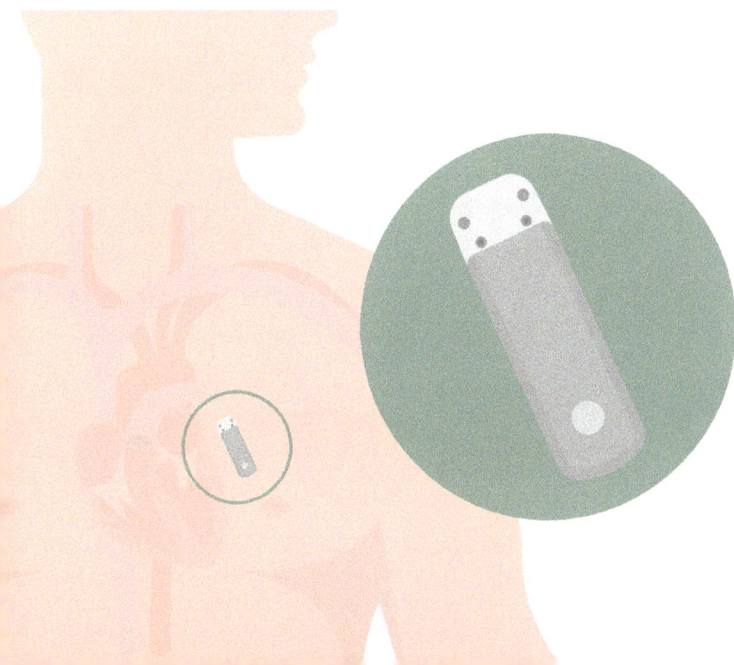

The company Neuralink is developing an implant to record brain activity and transmit data to a computer. It could allow a patient suffering from paralysis to control a keyboard and send text messages with their thoughts.

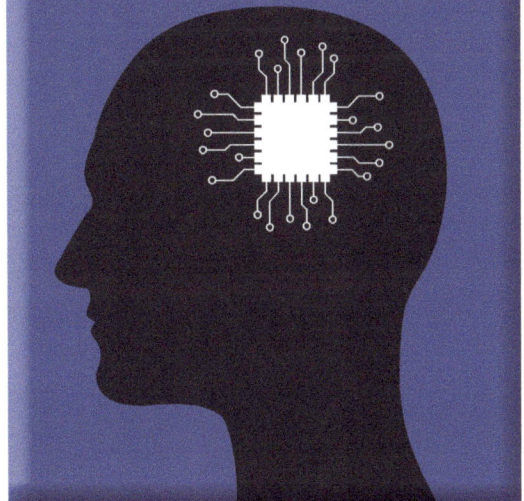

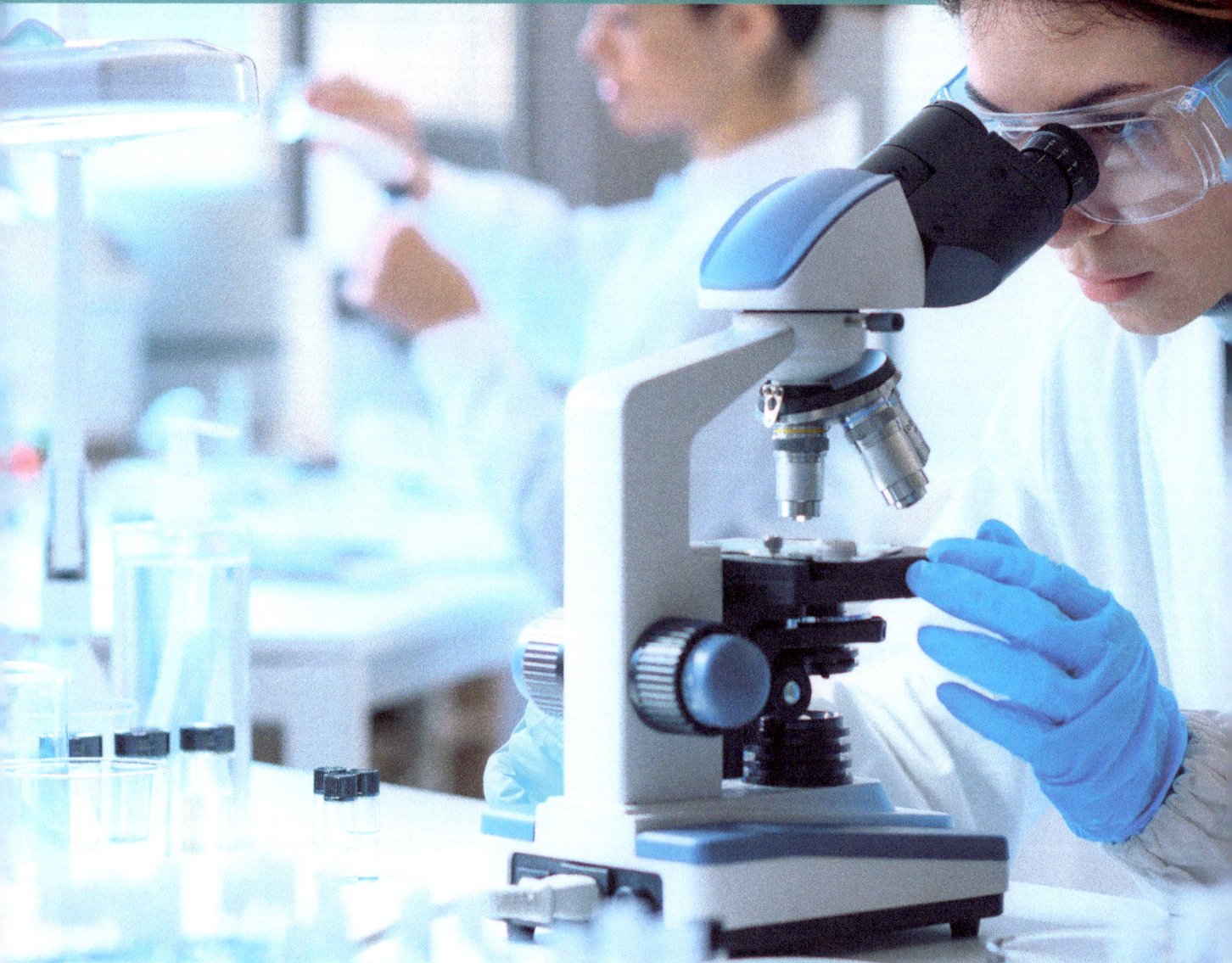

# 3 NANOMEDICINE

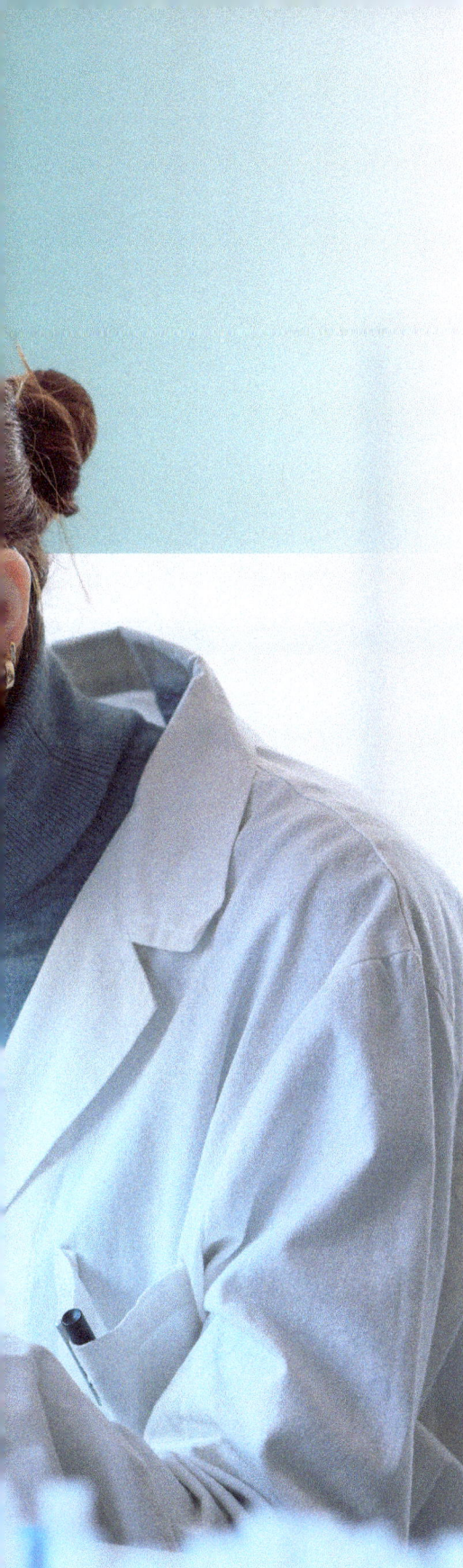

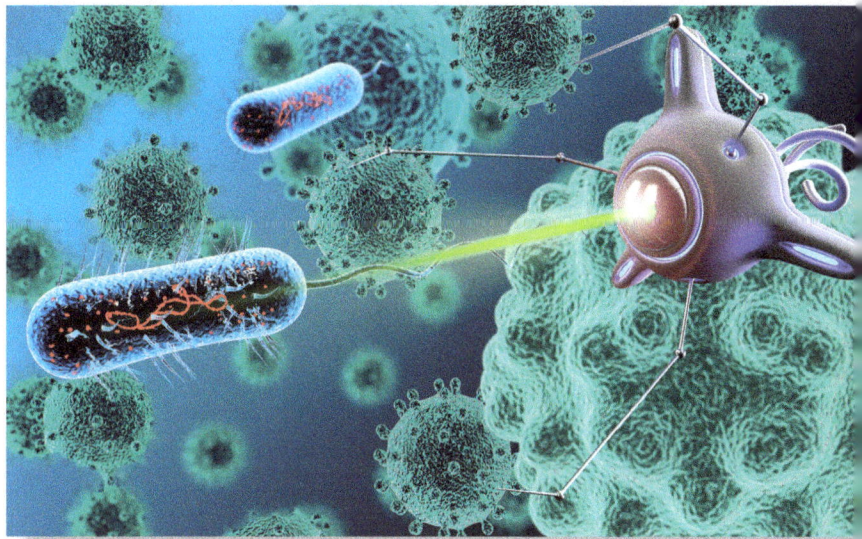

## TINY MEDICAL TOOLS

Think of a human hair. Now try to imagine something a thousand times thinner. That is the nanoscale. A hair is about 80,000 nanometers wide. Nanoparticles are between 1 and 100 nanometers in size. That's too small to be seen under all but the most powerful microscopes. The future of nanomedicine aims to use these tiny particles for medical purposes. Scientists plan to engineer nanoparticles to serve as precise tools inside the body. They may monitor the body's health, diagnose diseases, and deliver medicines.

Nanoscale medicine has many advantages. Nanoparticles can easily pass through cell membranes to deliver medicine. They can be coated with a material to prevent attack from the immune system. Nanomedicine is still a very young field. As it advances, techniques will become ever more sophisticated. It's possible to imagine a future where nanobots (nanoscale machines) roam our bodies carrying out repairs, collecting tissue samples, and destroying harmful germs.

# DIAGNOSIS

Some diseases begin as molecular changes that may not become symptoms for years. Medical nanoparticles are only slightly larger than molecules and can work as effective diagnostic tools. They can be coated with substances to bind or interact with *biomarkers* (disease identifiers). This can help doctors identify and treat diseases early—long before any symptoms appear. This improves the patient's chances of recovery or cure.

**Alzheimer's disease** mainly affects elderly people, causing a gradual mental decline. The first noticeable symptom is usually memory loss (forgetfulness). There is no cure, but the course of the disease may be slowed with treatment, especially if it is detected early. Nanomedicine may detect the disease by sensing microscopic changes in the brain before irreversible damage has begun. Medical nanoparticles are small enough to pass through the blood-brain barrier (BBB), a wall of cells that protects the brain and hampers diagnostic tests. Scientists want to design nanoparticles that cross the BBB and detect the microscopic biomarkers of Alzheimer's disease.

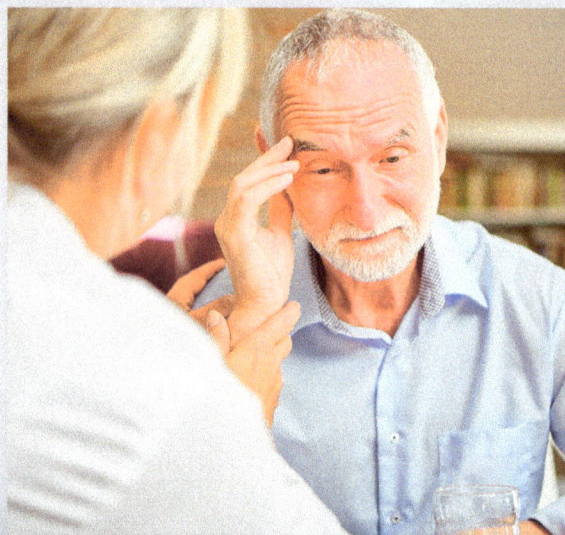

**Cancer.** Cancer cells spreading through the body produce biomarkers, which doctors can use to detect the disease. Early in the disease, there aren't enough biomarkers for easy detection. Engineered nanoparticles interact with cancer cells to induce them to increase biomarker production, so cancer can be detected earlier.

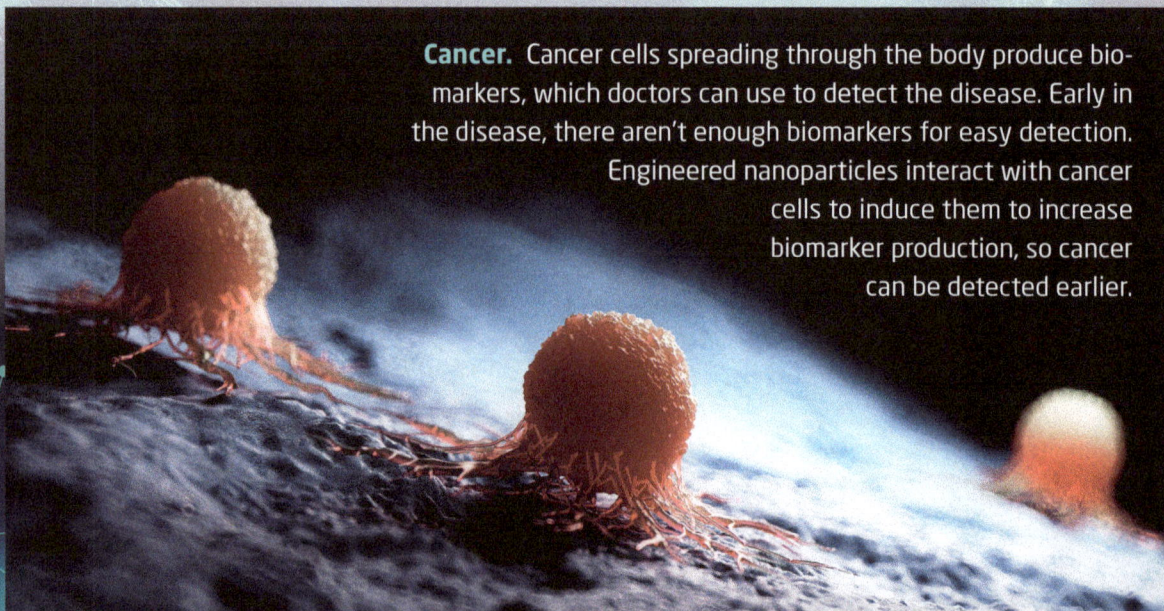

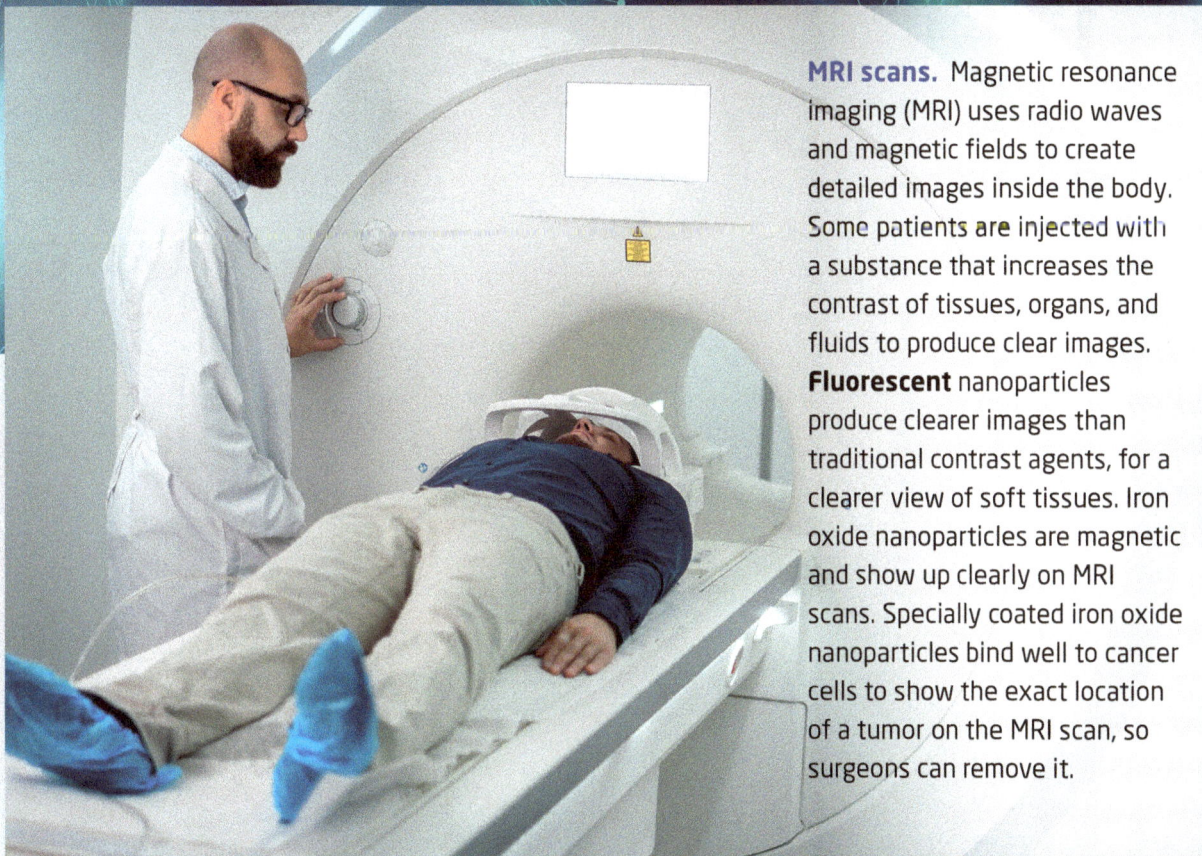

**MRI scans.** Magnetic resonance imaging (MRI) uses radio waves and magnetic fields to create detailed images inside the body. Some patients are injected with a substance that increases the contrast of tissues, organs, and fluids to produce clear images. **Fluorescent** nanoparticles produce clearer images than traditional contrast agents, for a clearer view of soft tissues. Iron oxide nanoparticles are magnetic and show up clearly on MRI scans. Specially coated iron oxide nanoparticles bind well to cancer cells to show the exact location of a tumor on the MRI scan, so surgeons can remove it.

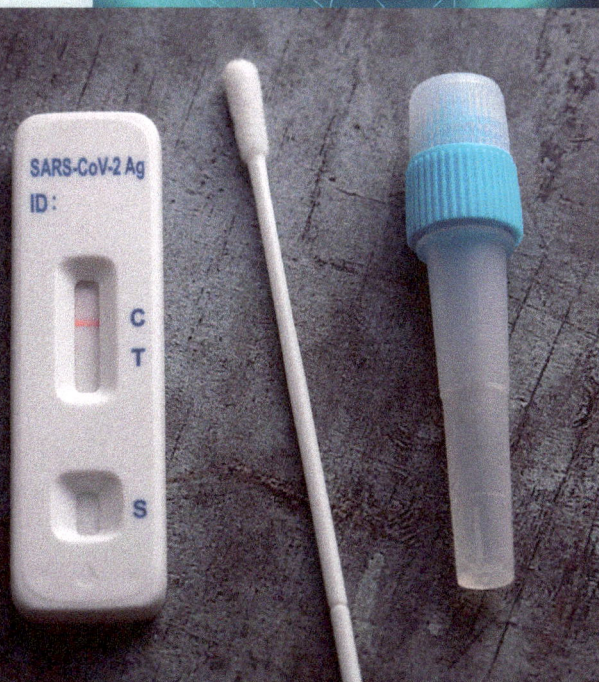

**Lateral flow tests.** (LFT's) diagnose infectious diseases. They consist of an absorbent pad at one end and a reading window at the other. When a saliva sample is added, it flows along the pad onto a special membrane. A colored line appears in the reading window if a disease biomarker is present. Most LFT's use gold nanoparticles, which stop the flow when biomarkers are contacted. These absorb green light and produce a red line to indicate a positive result when certain germs are detected. Researchers are exploring nanodiamonds for LFT's. Nanodiamond LFT's are less expensive to produce while improving the speed and accuracy of tests.

# TREATMENT

Nanomedicine has great potential to provide targeted, personalized medical treatment for a range of diseases and disorders. Nanoparticles can deliver medicines exactly where they are needed. This means a patient can take a lower dose of medicine, limiting harmful side effects. But medical nanoparticles may also have some risks. Experts worry that medical nanoparticles may persist in the body and cause unintended reactions or even cancer.

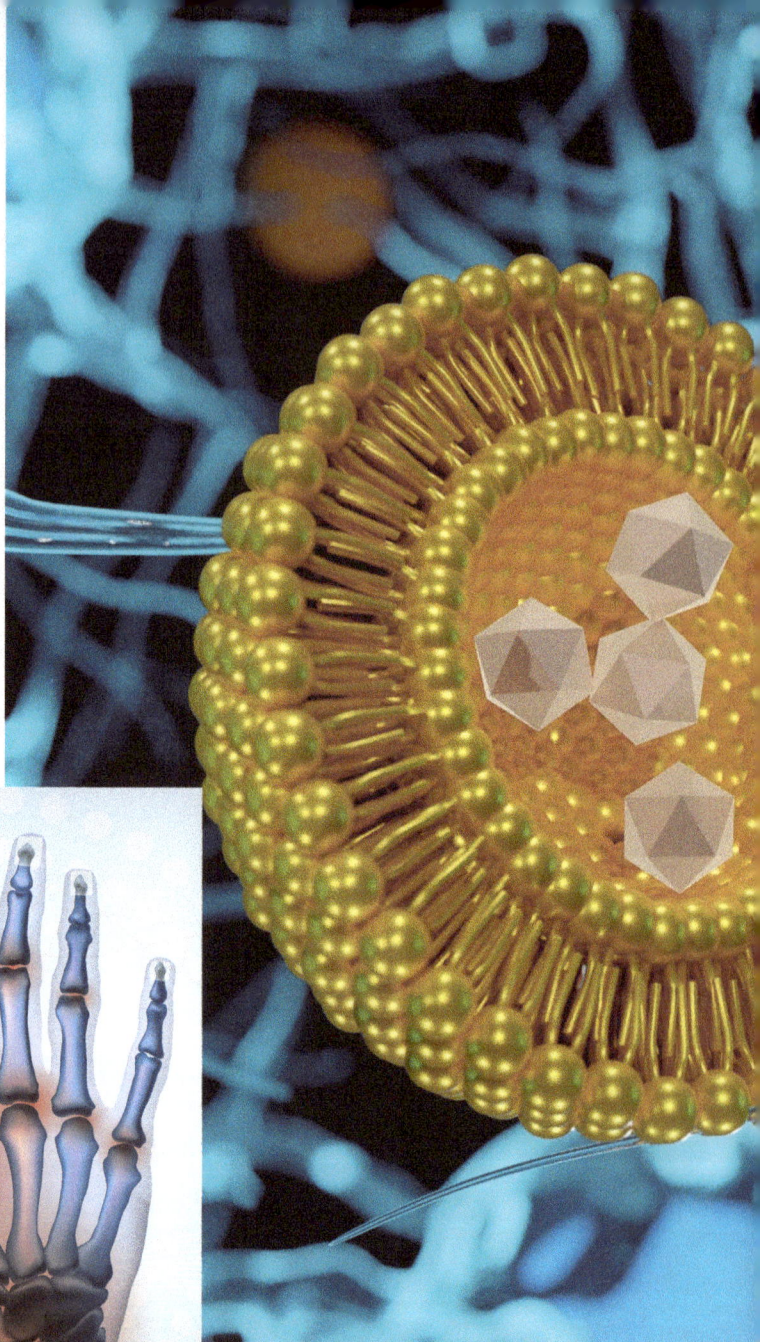

**Rheumatoid arthritis** is a disease where the body's immune system attacks the joints, causing painful inflammation. A project named NANOFOL has researched treatments using engineered nanoparticles 100–400 nanometers in width. The nanoparticles are coated with a chemical to bind with and disable macrophages (germ-killing cells of the immune system). Other nanoparticles could deliver anti-inflammatory medicines to the joints.

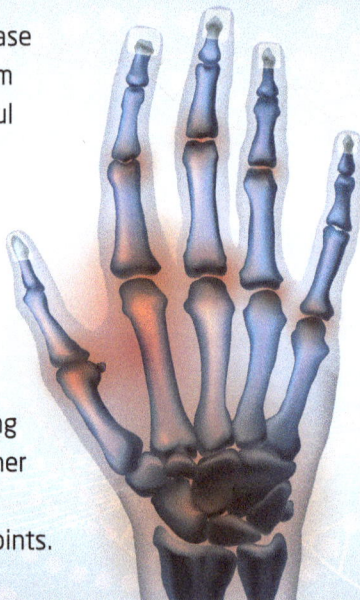

**Diabetes.** Many people with diabetes must inject insulin to control blood glucose (sugar) levels. This is often inconvenient and painful. Taking an insulin pill would be easier, but insulin is destroyed by stomach acid. In 2021, a team of scientists in China and the UK researched the idea of coating insulin molecules in a layer of nanoparticles to protect the vital medicine from stomach acid and promote its absorption.

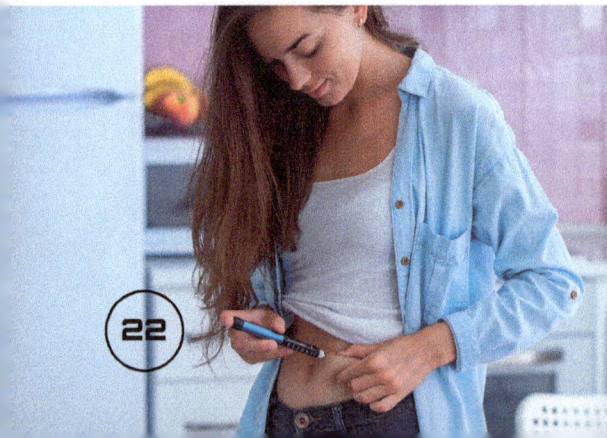

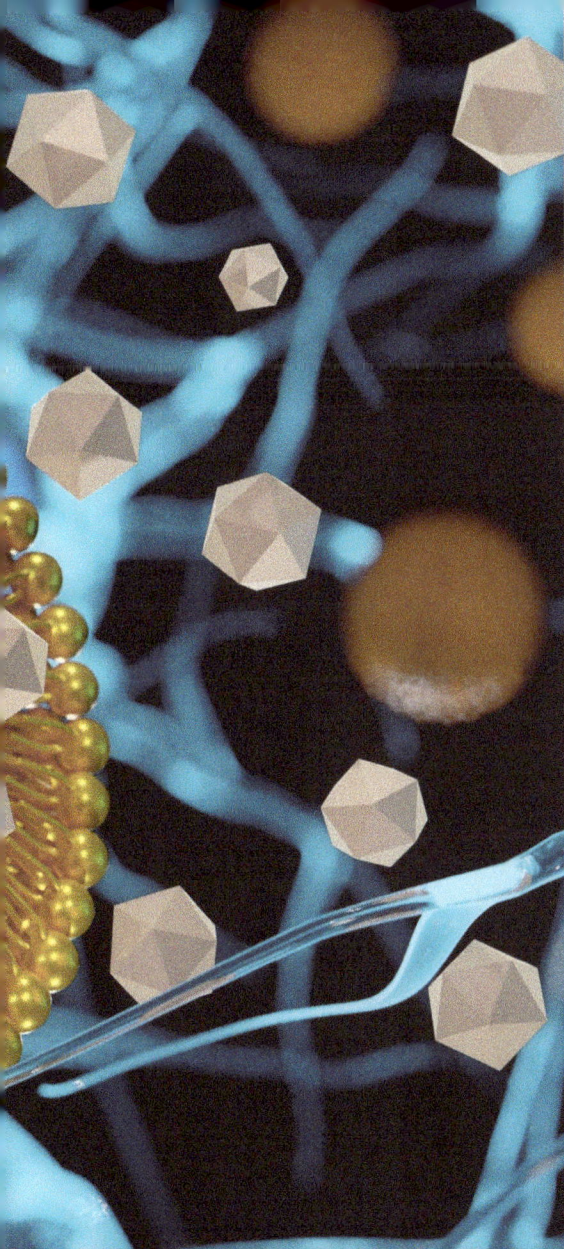

**Eye treatments.** Nanoparticles in eye drops can deliver medicines for eye disorders. Engineered nanoparticles can form a medicated gel to treat eye inflammations. Other medical nanoparticles made from lipids (fats) can deliver a molecule named myriocin precisely to the retina (the layer at the back of the eye). This molecule reduces degeneration of the retina's *photoreceptors* (light-sensitive cells).

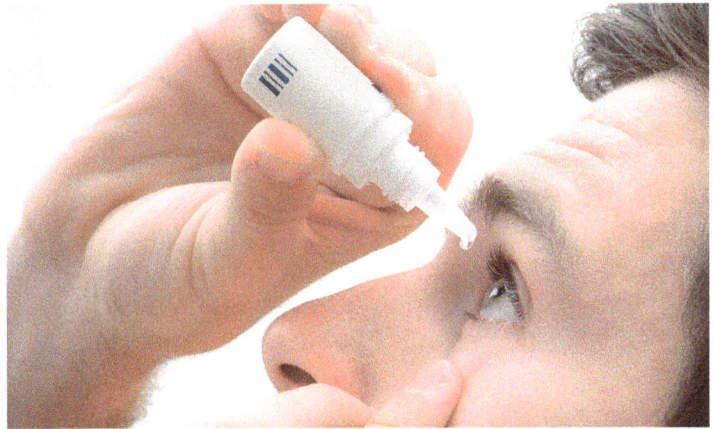

**Nanobots.** Medical nanoscale robots, or nanobots, will one day propel themselves through our bodies and heal us from the inside. Scientists from the University of California, USA, plan to create tiny beads of magnesium or titanium propelled by bubbles of hydrogen that will move themselves to a stomach ulcer, where they will release medicine and then dissolve. Researchers at Drexel University, Pennsylvania, USA, are developing corkscrew-shaped nanobots made of a chain of iron oxide beads. These will be injected into the bloodstream to unblock arteries by drilling through and breaking up fatty deposits. A team at a university in Zurich, Switzerland, is developing a magnetic nanobot that can be injected into the eye. They hope that one day surgeons will be able to perform delicate operations by manipulating the nanobot with a magnetic field.

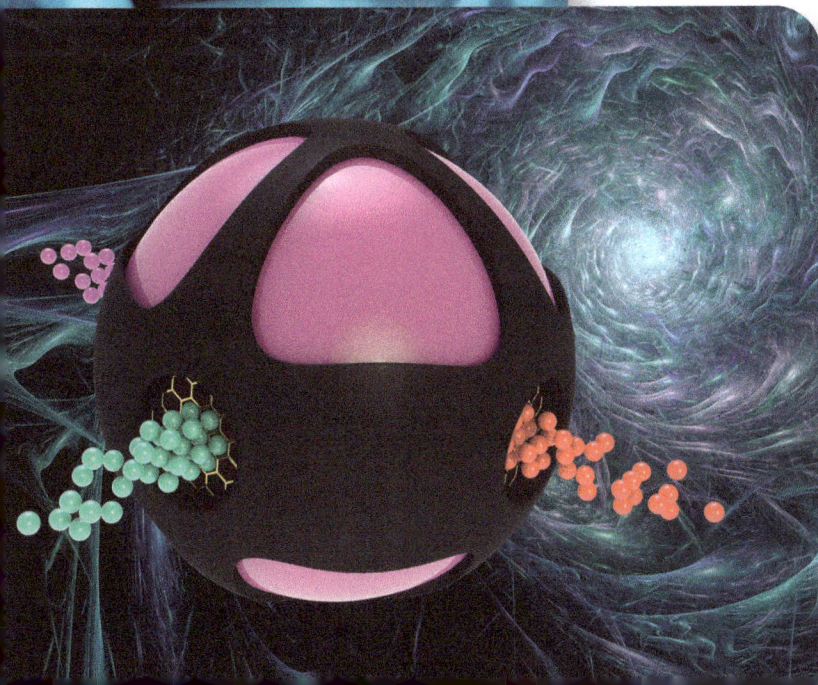

# 4 ARTIFICIAL INTELLIGENCE

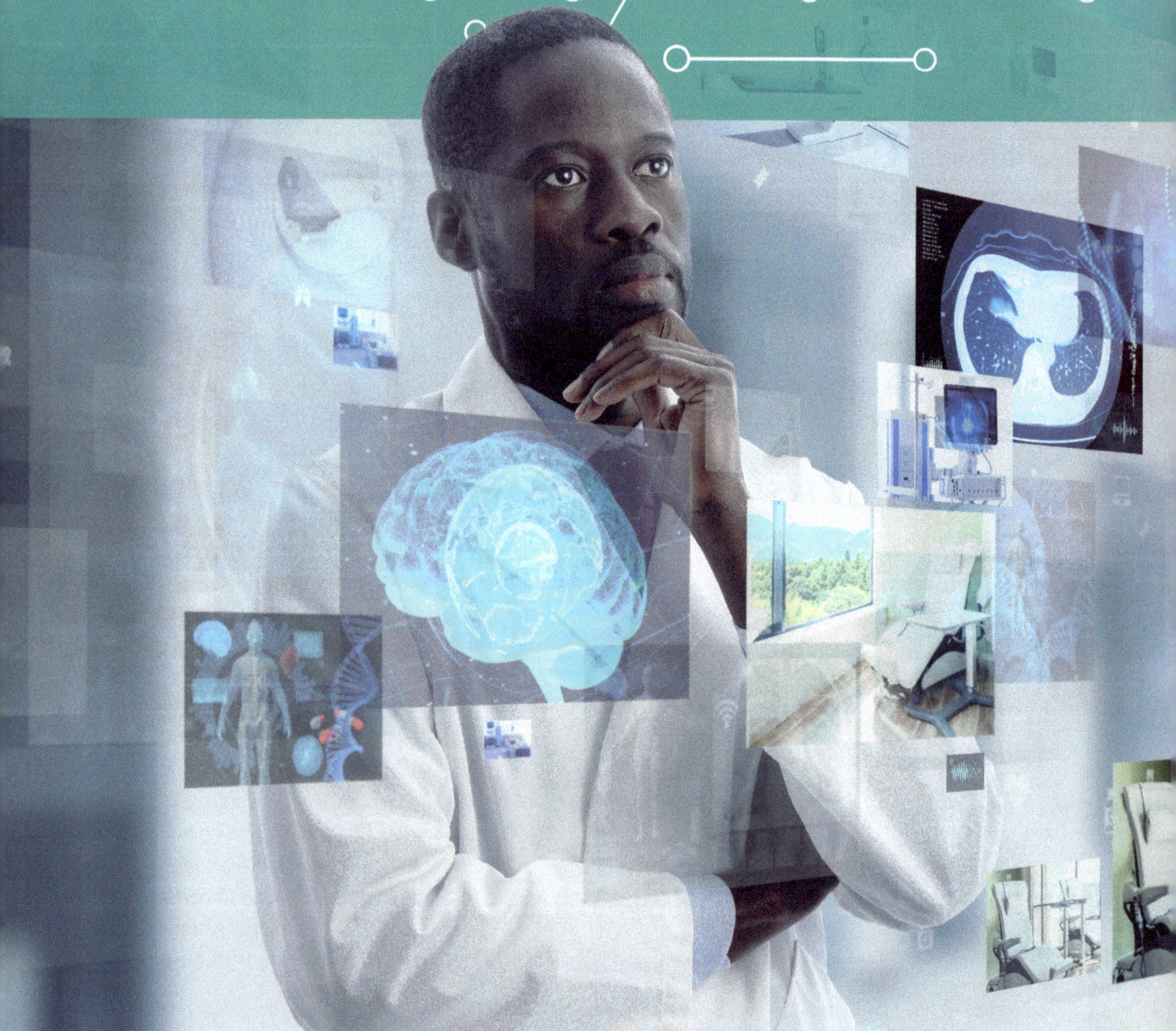

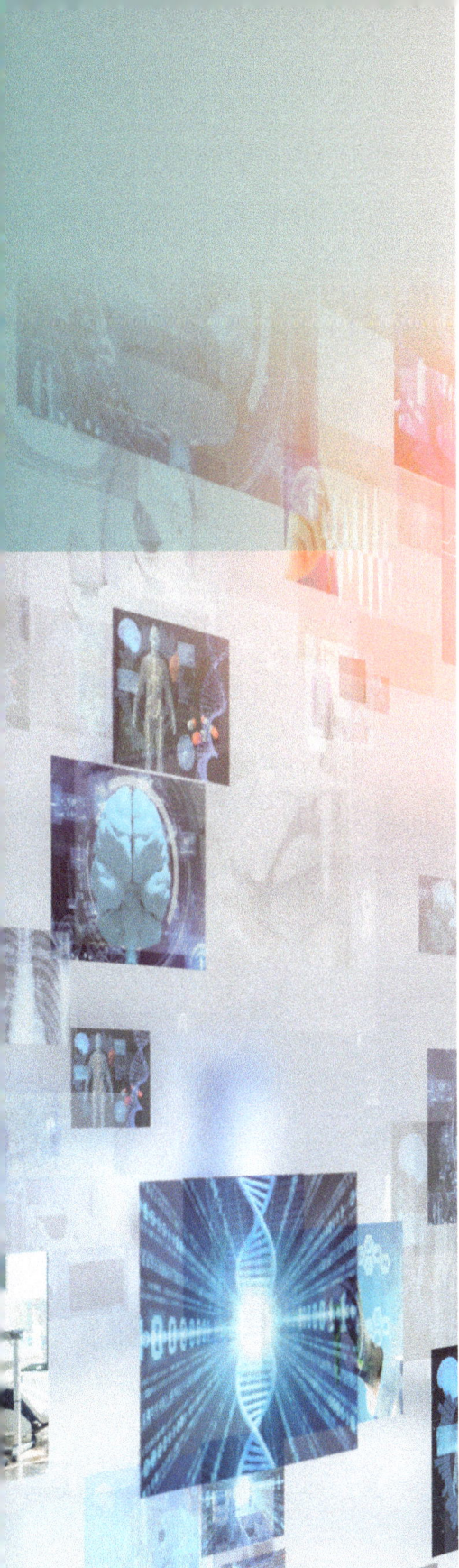

# A QUIET REVOLUTION

Today, an invisible labor force works in the background of the world's hospitals, clinics, and medical laboratories. Intelligent computer programs are busy helping diagnose diseases, analyze scans, and research new medicines. The emergence of artificial intelligence (AI) in medicine has been a quiet revolution—and it's only just beginning.

An AI algorithm is a set of rules written in code a computer can understand. A neural network is one kind of algorithm that can "learn" as it operates. An AI neural network can analyze MRI scans and search for a tumor. The algorithm compares thousands of similar MRI scans to "learn" what to look for.

AI programs are revolutionizing medicine today. AI can do jobs in minutes that would take humans hours or days to perform. AI relieves hardworking medical technicians of routine tasks, such as managing data, designing treatments, ordering supplies, monitoring patients, and answering basic questions from patients and the public. AI programs work tirelessly and efficiently without a break. The programs help reduce health care costs and medical errors. They help improve patient safety and free health care workers to spend more time engaging with patients.

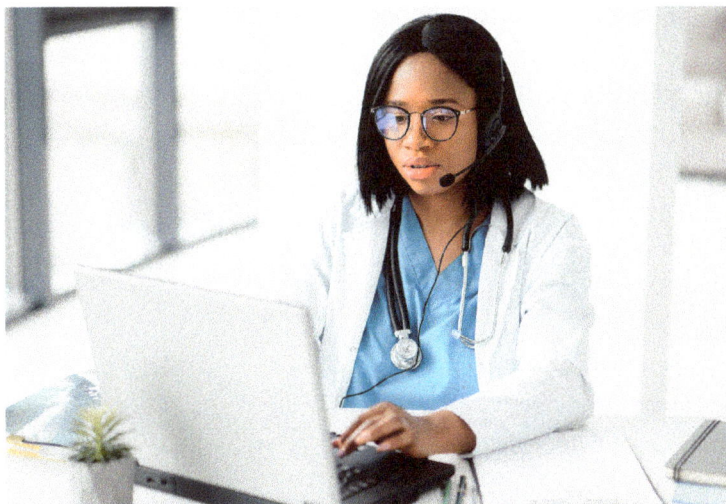

# DIAGNOSIS AND TREATMENT

We all rely on our previous experience to make decisions. Doctors are no different. Their experience with symptoms and successful treatments guides patient care. But personal experience can sometimes be misleading. An AI program can draw upon vastly more data than any single doctor. It can compare symptoms to similar cases from all over the world. Doctors know that different diseases can have similar symptoms. Experienced doctors can distinguish symptoms and diagnose various conditions. Today, medical AI can compete with the most experienced doctors around.

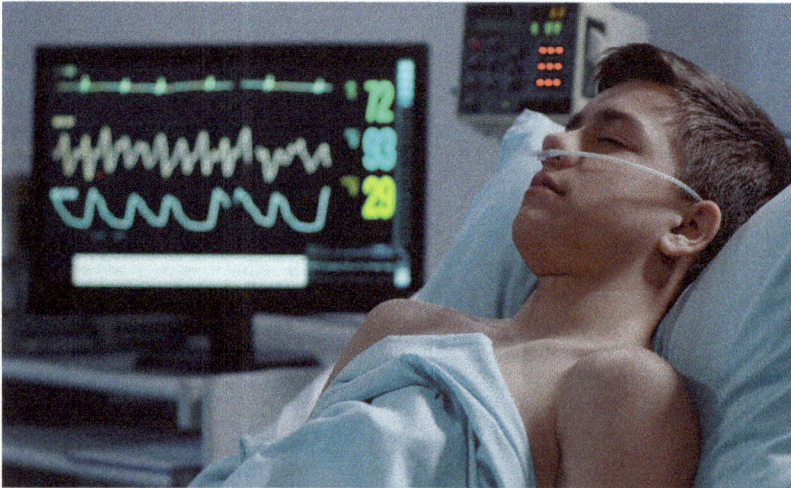

**Hospitals.** Today, AI helps hospital personnel treat the thousands of people who pass through every day. AI is used to help prioritize patients based on the severity of their condition. AI can speed up diagnosis at critical moments and monitor patient vital signs around the clock. And it alerts medical staff if anything goes wrong.

**Mental health.** Woebot is an AI **chatbot** that helps patients with depression and anxiety (uneasy thoughts). Woebot engages in empathetic conversations, suggests mood-improving activities, monitors a patient's state of mind, and helps patients treat their symptoms. An AI algorithm called Ellipsis Health can analyze a patient's voice and speech patterns for signs of emotional stress, anxiety, and depression.

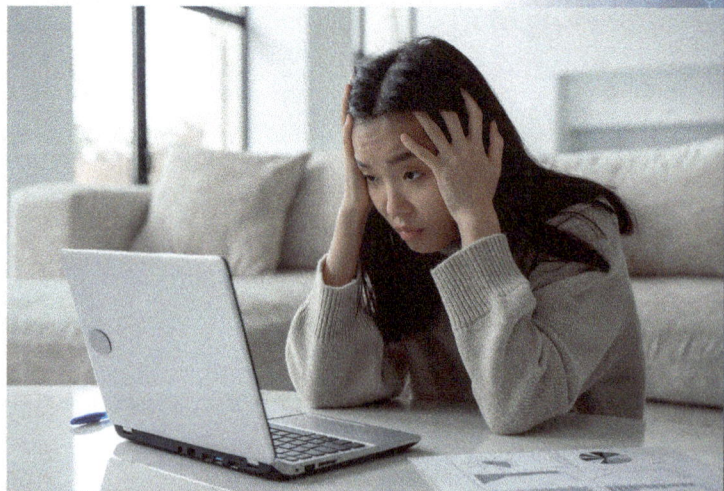

**Natural language processing.** Augmedix uses AI neural networks trained to understand spoken language from doctor-patient conversations and convert them into medical notes in real time. An AI-powered smartphone app named Babylon Health can listen to a user describe their symptoms and offer them health advice or match them to a relevant doctor. Corti is a medical app that listens in on emergency calls and analyzes the caller's voice and background noises. Comparing this to historical data, it can alert EMS if the neural network program identifies a medical emergency, such as a heart attack in progress.

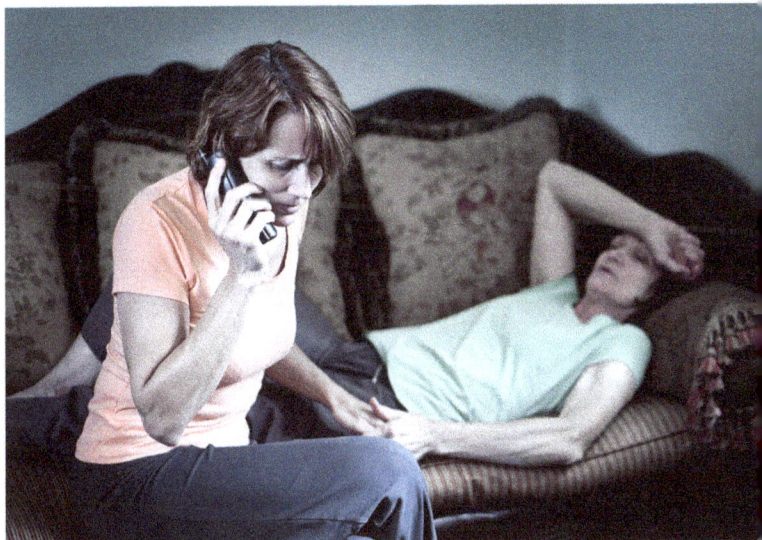

**Mapping human health.** Doctors usually see patients only after they get sick, so we know little about how diseases begin. Thanks to AI, that will all change. Verily Life Sciences launched Project Baseline, which aims to map human health over time. The project collects years of medical data from thousands of participants from diverse backgrounds. Project Baseline subjects wear wrist sensors, submit surveys, provide clinical data and imaging, and self-report their health status. Verily algorithms analyze, evaluate, and organize this information into a comprehensive database. The goal is to help medical professionals better understand the transition from health to disease and identify risk factors for disease.

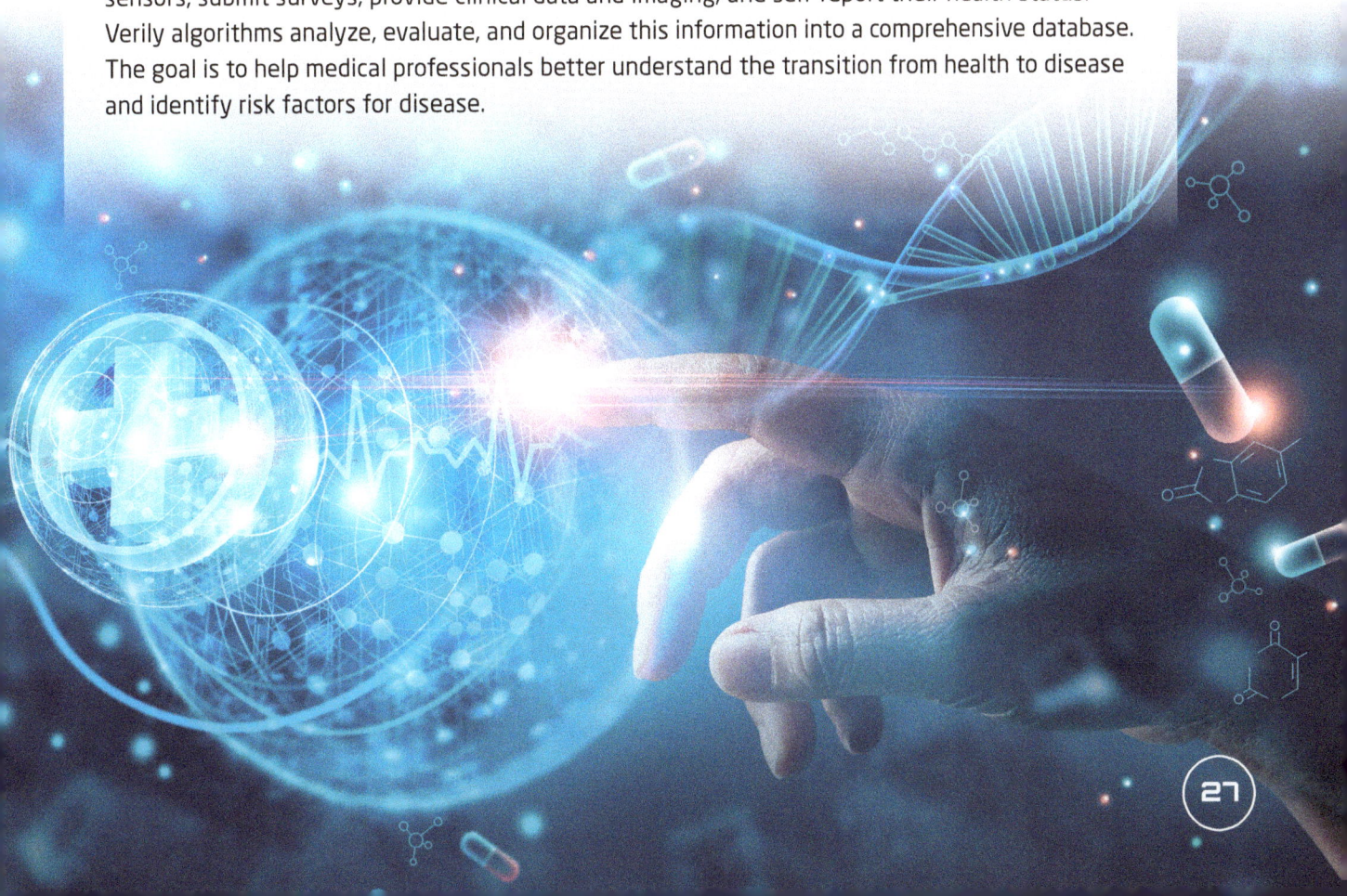

# MEDICAL SCANS

Advances in medical imaging technology allow doctors to obtain remarkably detailed views of the human body. Today, doctors use AI tools to scan medical images for tiny disease markers that the trained eye can miss. AI scan analysis is used to diagnose medical conditions and as a tool for treating them. For example, an algorithm can monitor successive tumor scans so that doctors can determine if a therapy is working or should be changed.

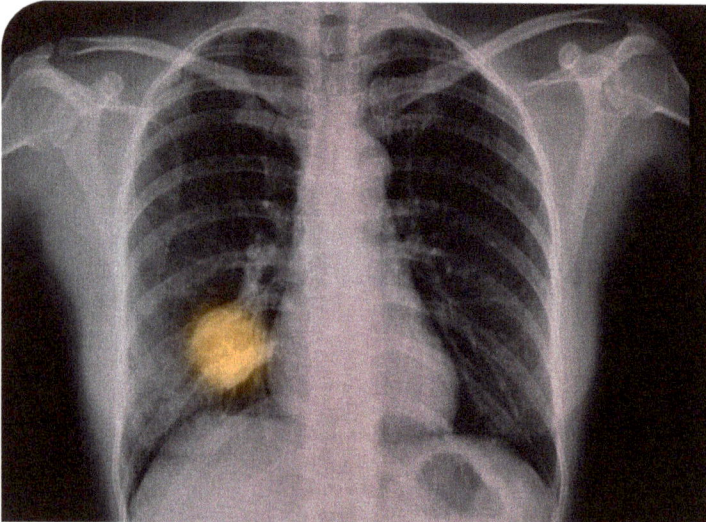

**Monitoring tumors.** AI can help determine the status of a tumor following medical treatment. A scanning technique called optoacoustic imaging turns light into sound signals. **Lasers** aimed at a tumor cause its cells to vibrate and generate sound waves. An algorithm analyzes changes in the sound waves to determine which parts of the tumor are alive and growing and which are not.

**Imaging brain activity.** Scientists have long sought an imaging technology that can accurately map the electrical activity of the brain. MRI scans are highly detailed but not fast enough to capture the rapid changes in brain activity. Electroencephalograms (EEG's) can capture brain activity but lack the resolution of an MRI. An AI neural network developed at Carnegie Mellon University, Pennsylvania, USA, could provide a solution. It can convert EEG signals into detailed images, helping doctors diagnose diseases and plan brain surgery.

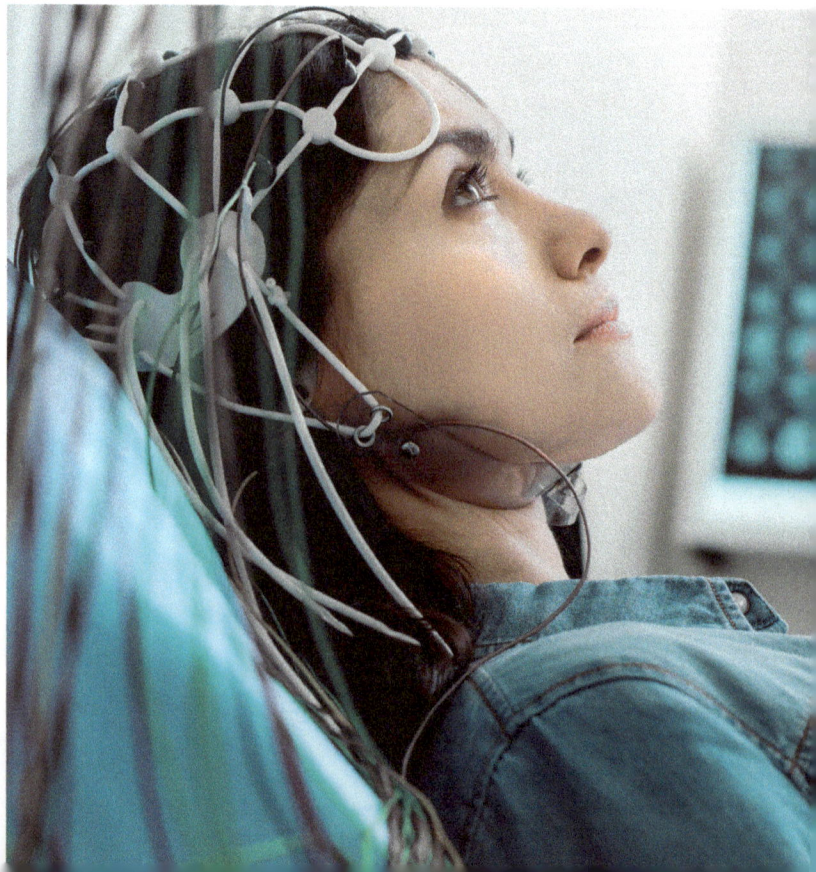

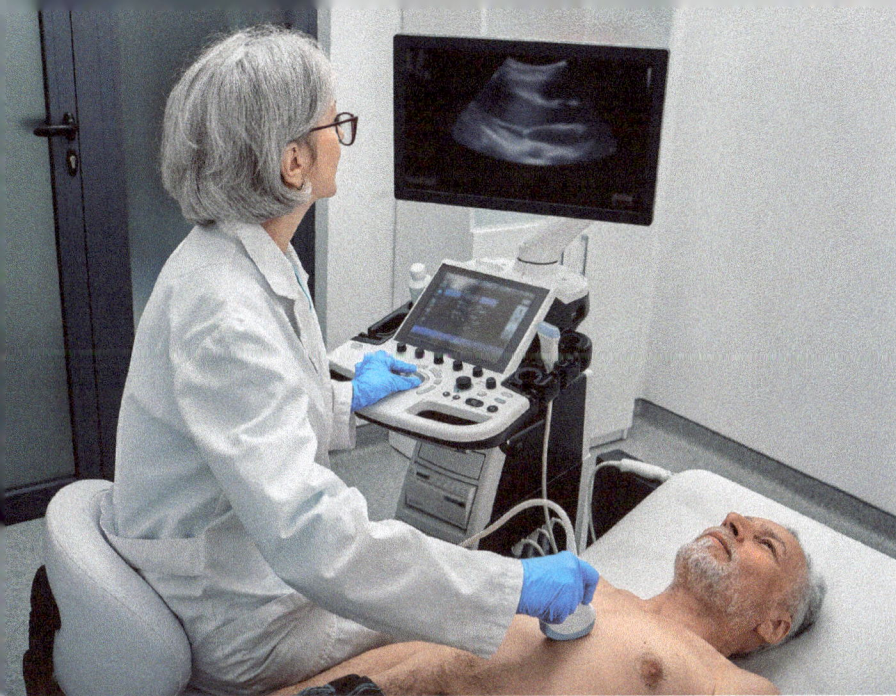

**Heart abnormalities.** AI tools are better than humans at detecting heart abnormalities by analyzing medical scans. AI tools precisely measure the enlargement of heart chambers, thickening of the heart muscle, or changes in blood flow through the heart. AI algorithms compare thousands of similar scans to spot and flag any measurement that falls outside of normal parameters.

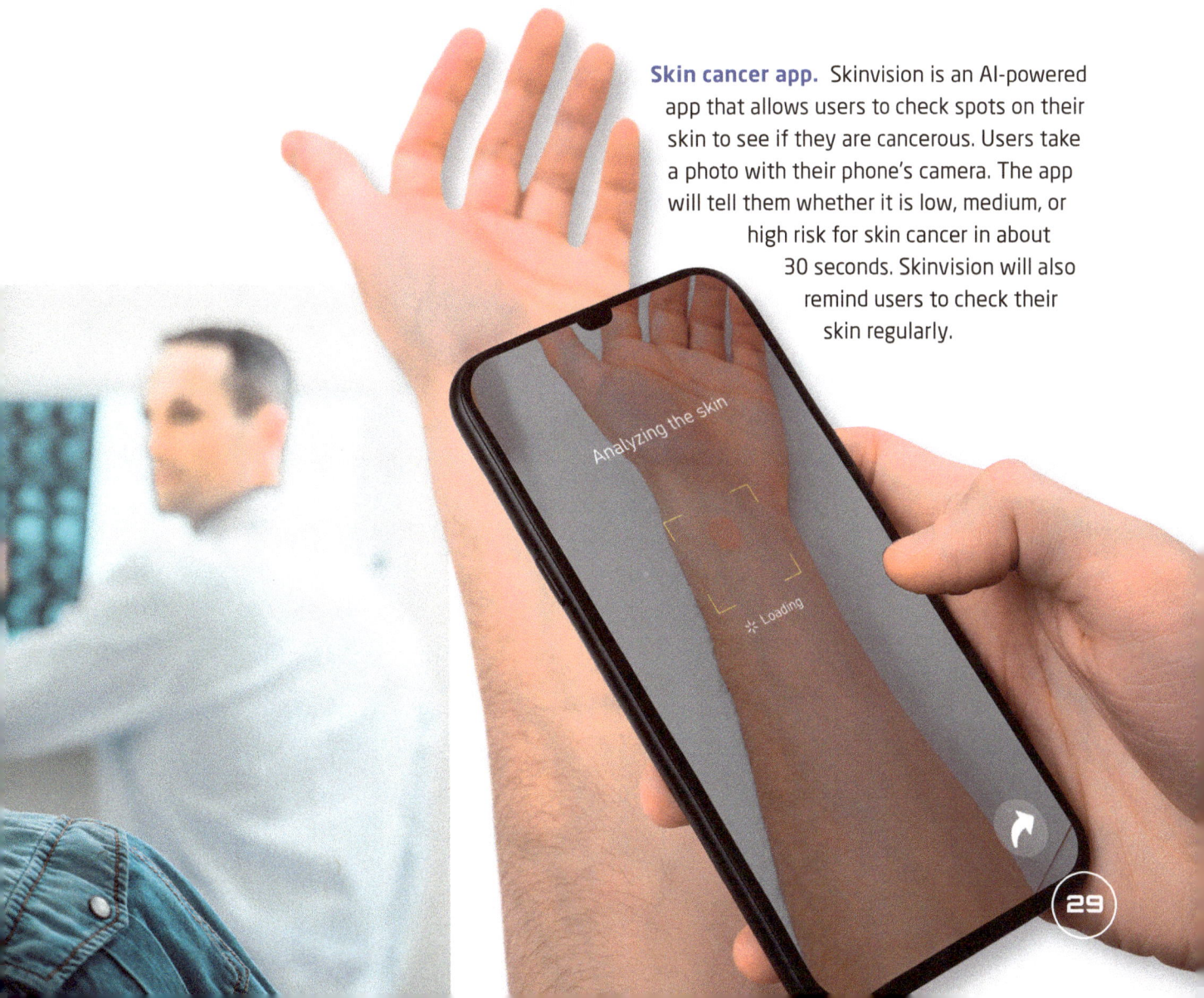

**Skin cancer app.** Skinvision is an AI-powered app that allows users to check spots on their skin to see if they are cancerous. Users take a photo with their phone's camera. The app will tell them whether it is low, medium, or high risk for skin cancer in about 30 seconds. Skinvision will also remind users to check their skin regularly.

Analyzing the skin

Loading

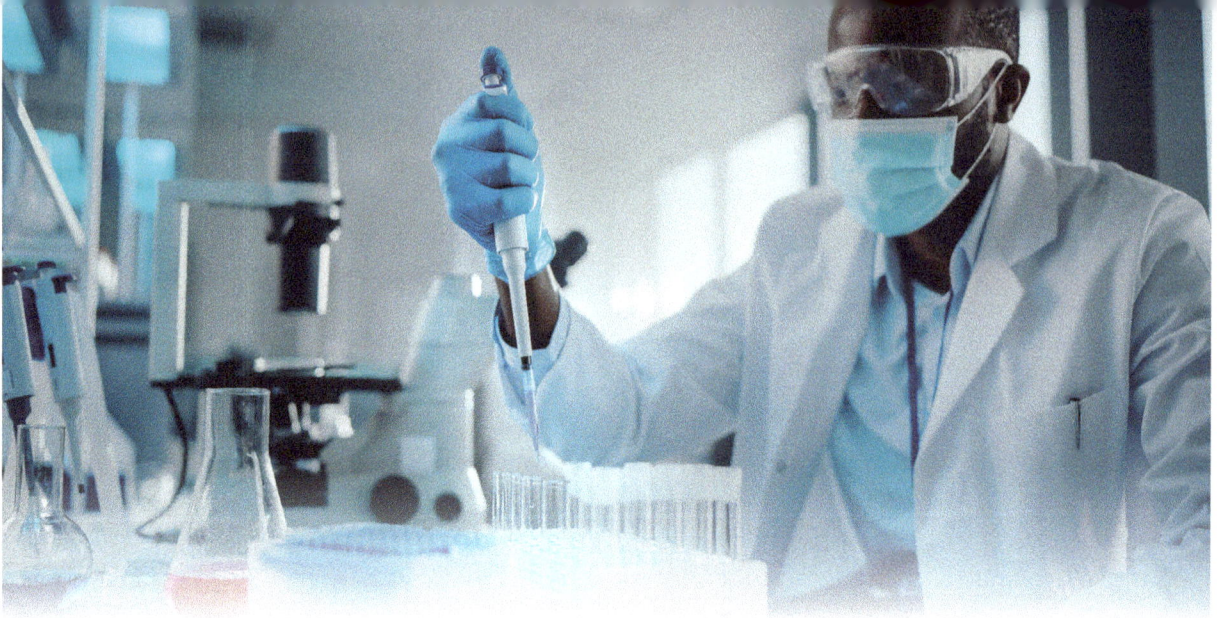

# RESEARCHING NEW MEDICINES

It takes 12 to 14 years and billions of dollars to bring a new medication to market. Much of this time and money is swallowed up by the research process. For every drug sold in a pharmacy, millions of others may have been tested and then rejected as unsuitable. AI can greatly streamline this process, helping reduce the time and cost of developing new medicines.

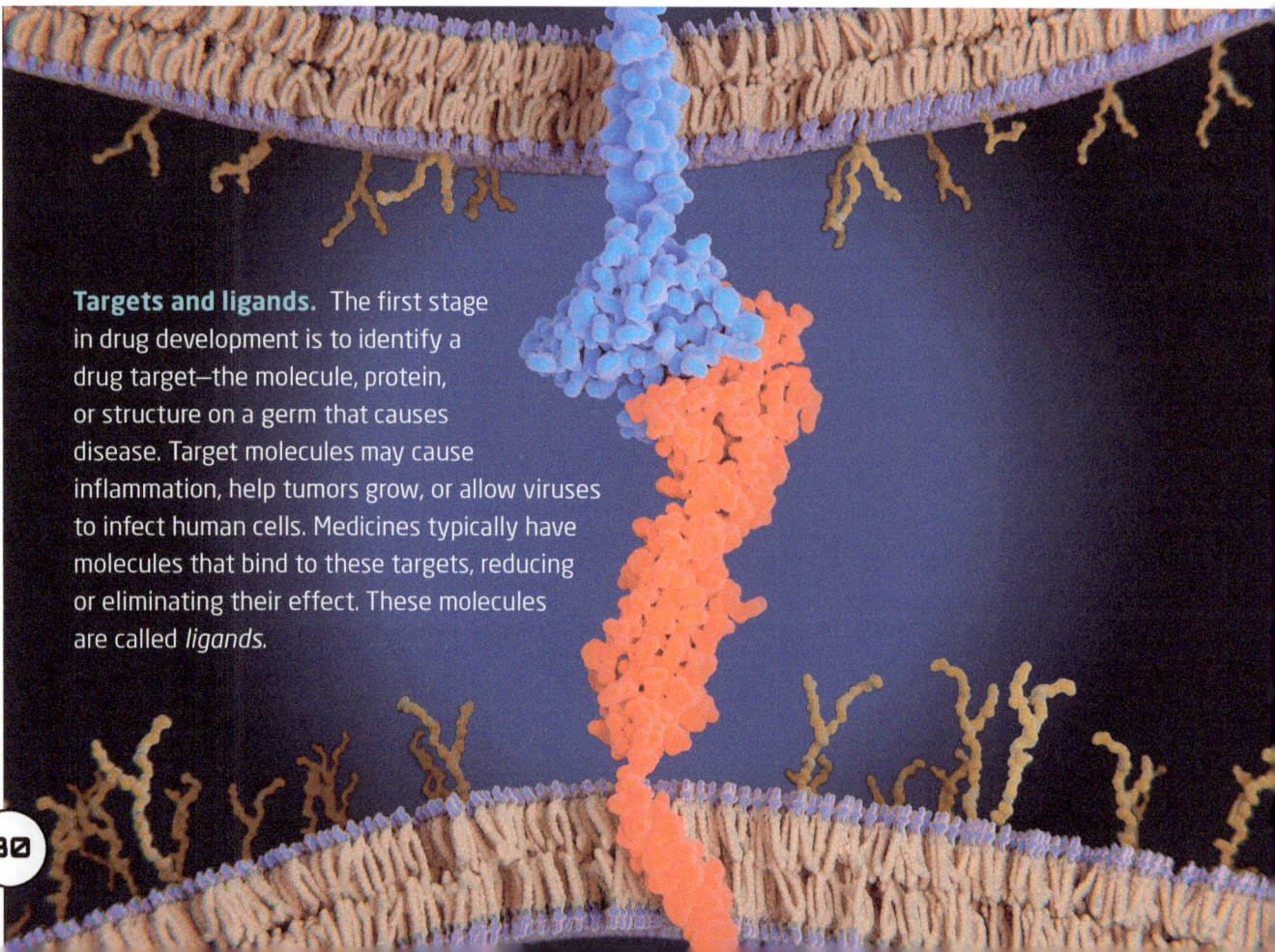

**Targets and ligands.** The first stage in drug development is to identify a drug target—the molecule, protein, or structure on a germ that causes disease. Target molecules may cause inflammation, help tumors grow, or allow viruses to infect human cells. Medicines typically have molecules that bind to these targets, reducing or eliminating their effect. These molecules are called *ligands*.

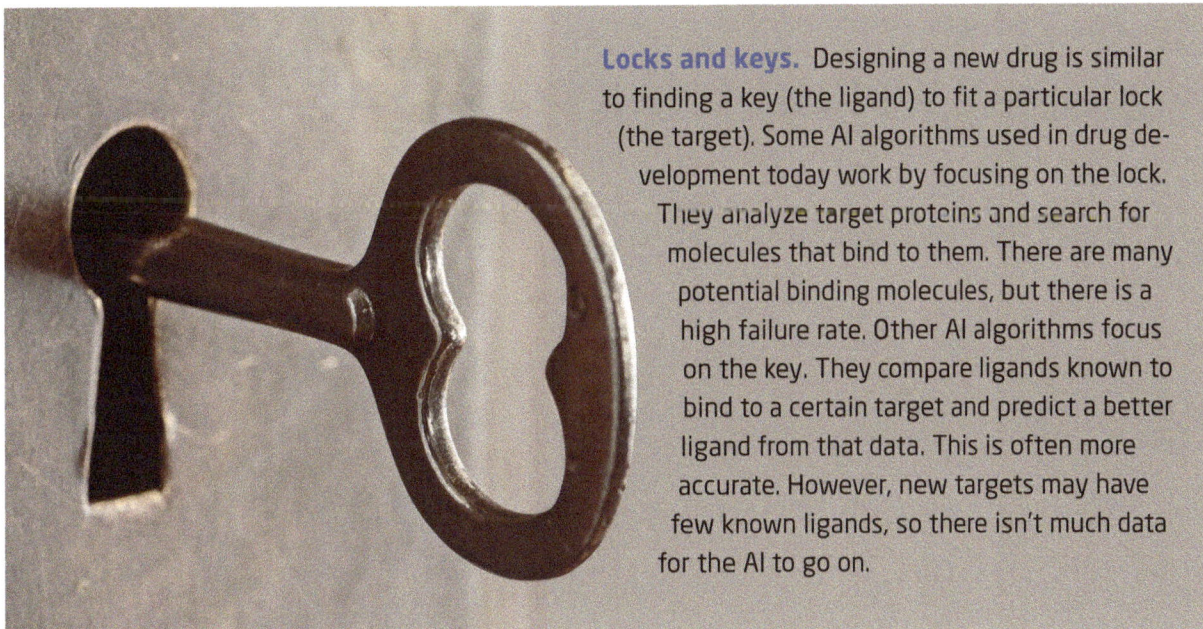

**Locks and keys.** Designing a new drug is similar to finding a key (the ligand) to fit a particular lock (the target). Some AI algorithms used in drug development today work by focusing on the lock. They analyze target proteins and search for molecules that bind to them. There are many potential binding molecules, but there is a high failure rate. Other AI algorithms focus on the key. They compare ligands known to bind to a certain target and predict a better ligand from that data. This is often more accurate. However, new targets may have few known ligands, so there isn't much data for the AI to go on.

**Convolutional neural networks.** A company named Atomwise has tried a new approach, using a convolutional neural network (CNN). This type of AI learns complex concepts by combining many smaller pieces of information. A CNN would learn to recognize cats by first learning basic features such as fur, whiskers, eyes, and tail, and combining them. Proteins and ligands can also be understood as combinations of more basic features, such as molecules of hydrogen and carbon. Atomwise's CNN is showing promise as a powerful tool for discovering new drugs.

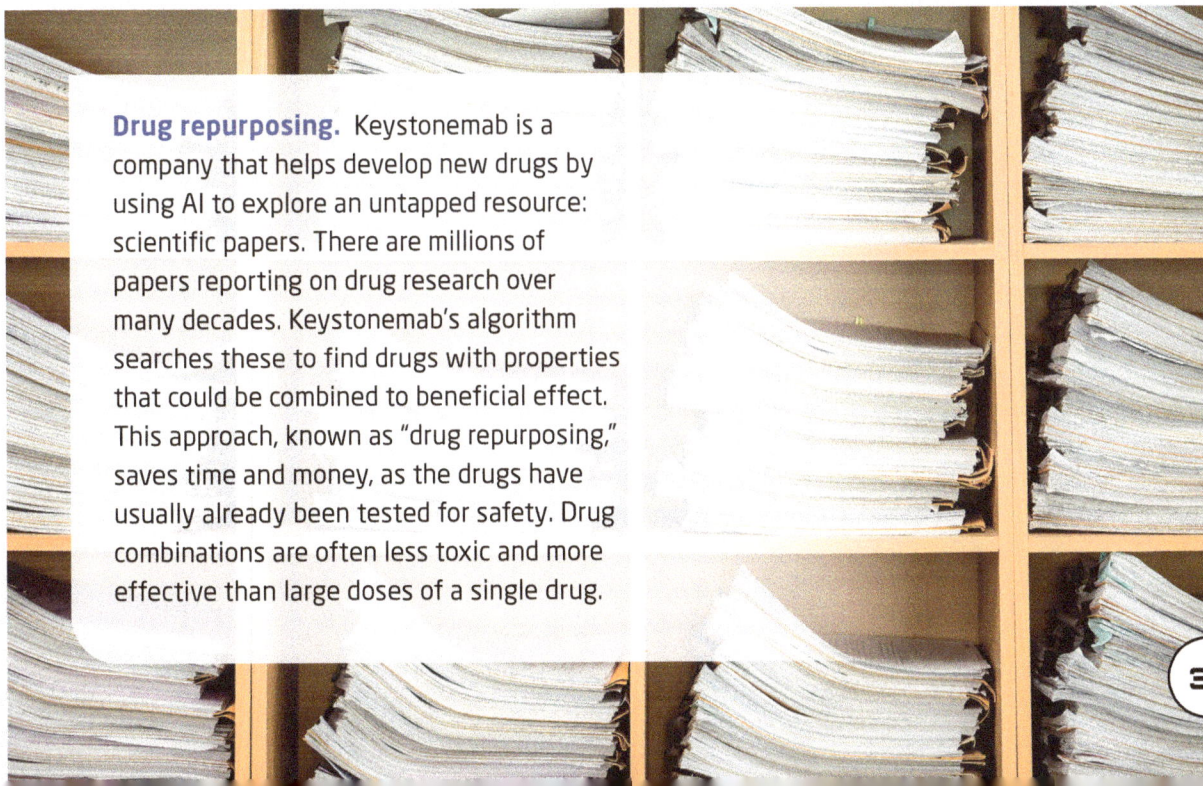

**Drug repurposing.** Keystonemab is a company that helps develop new drugs by using AI to explore an untapped resource: scientific papers. There are millions of papers reporting on drug research over many decades. Keystonemab's algorithm searches these to find drugs with properties that could be combined to beneficial effect. This approach, known as "drug repurposing," saves time and money, as the drugs have usually already been tested for safety. Drug combinations are often less toxic and more effective than large doses of a single drug.

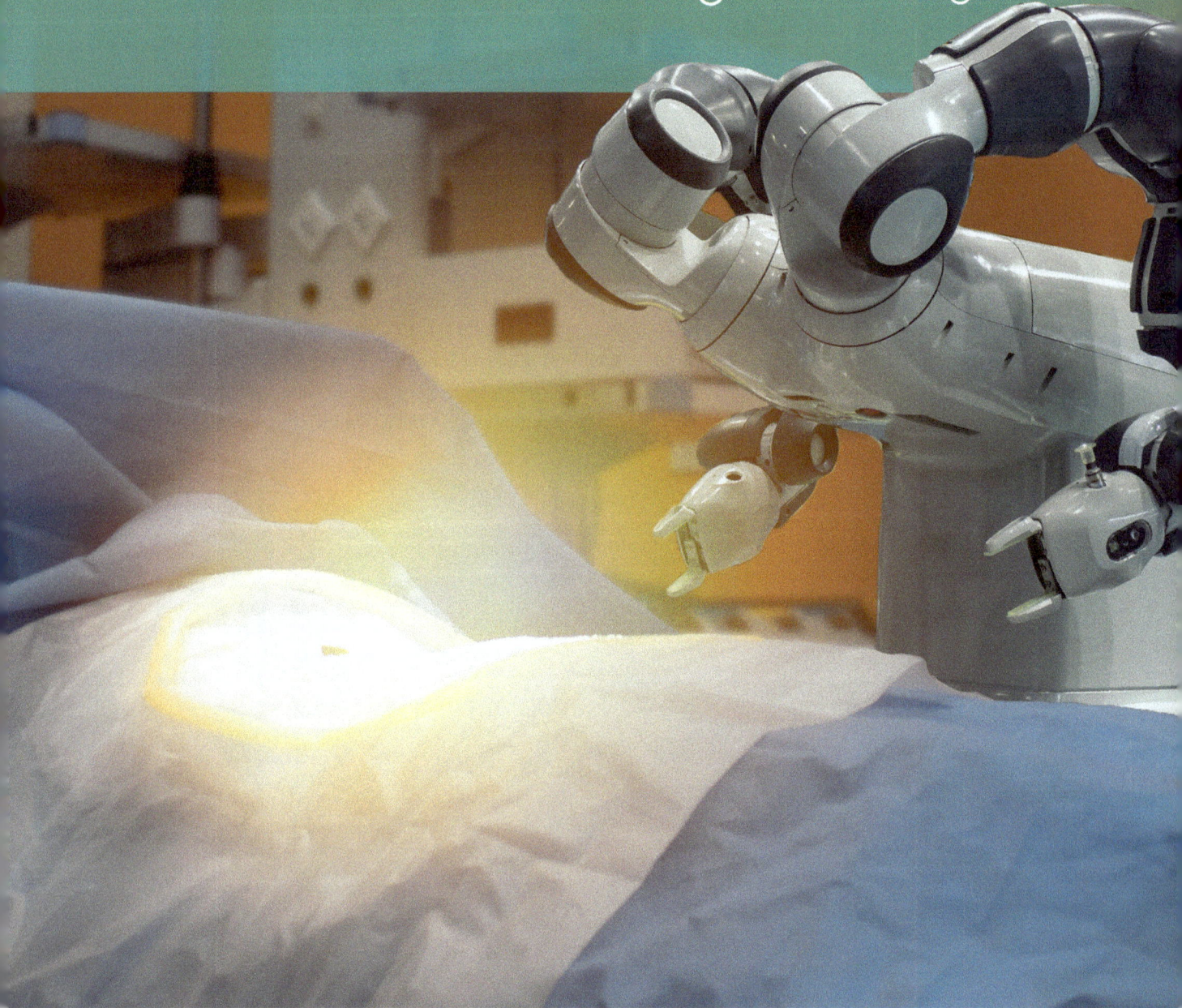

# 5 ROBOTICS

# THE RISE OF ROBOTIC ASSISTANTS

Robots are an increasing presence in hospitals and other medical settings. Thanks to advances in AI, computer vision, and engineering, their role is expanding all the time.

Robots are ideal surgical assistants because they are dextrous (skilled), flexible, and steady. They also take on the routine, arduous, or risky jobs that human hospital workers once had to do. Robots today deliver supplies, clean and disinfect hospital rooms, and move beds and patients, allowing medical staff to focus more on patient care. Robots are used in medical research labs to automate repetitive, high-volume, and time-consuming tasks.

Robots cut the costs of health care, increase safety in hospitals, and improve the quality of patient care. But these benefits come with some risks. Robots can malfunction. They may suffer mechanical or software failures and endanger patients and staff. Nevertheless, robots are likely to become a common sight in hospital wards, operating rooms, and corridors.

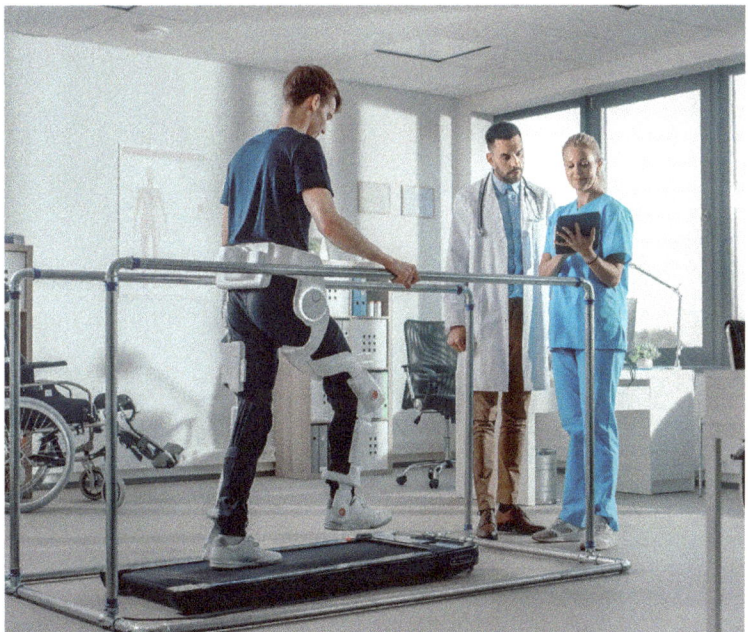

# SURGICAL ROBOTS

Robots have been assisting surgeons for many years. One robotic system named da Vinci has been in use since 2000. By the end of 2021, it had assisted in more than ten million operations around the world. Robots help surgeons work quickly and accurately during complex operations. They assist in minimally invasive surgery by manipulating tiny surgical instruments through small *incisions* (cuts) in the flesh.

**Smaller incisions.** In traditional surgery, surgeons must make a large incision in the patient's body to accommodate their hands and fingers. Robots equipped with small, narrow instruments work with tiny incisions. This reduces blood loss and the risk of infection, so patients recover faster. After an incision is made, the robot locks itself in place, creating a stable platform for surgery. A human surgeon seated at a nearby console manipulates the instruments via remote control.

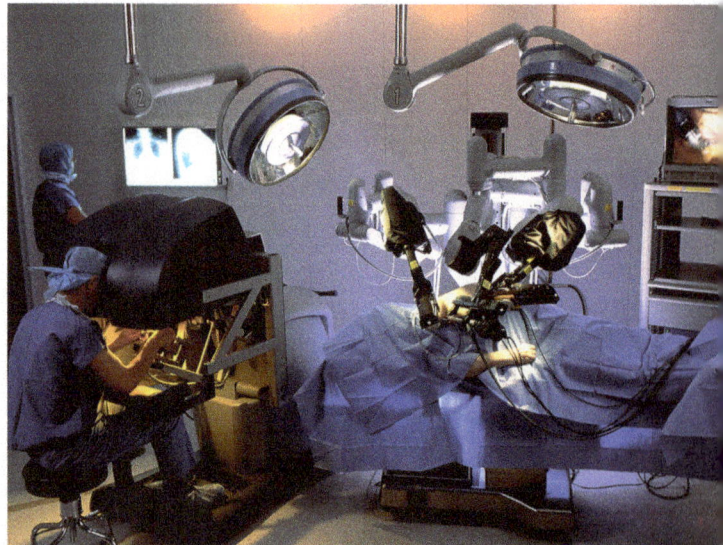

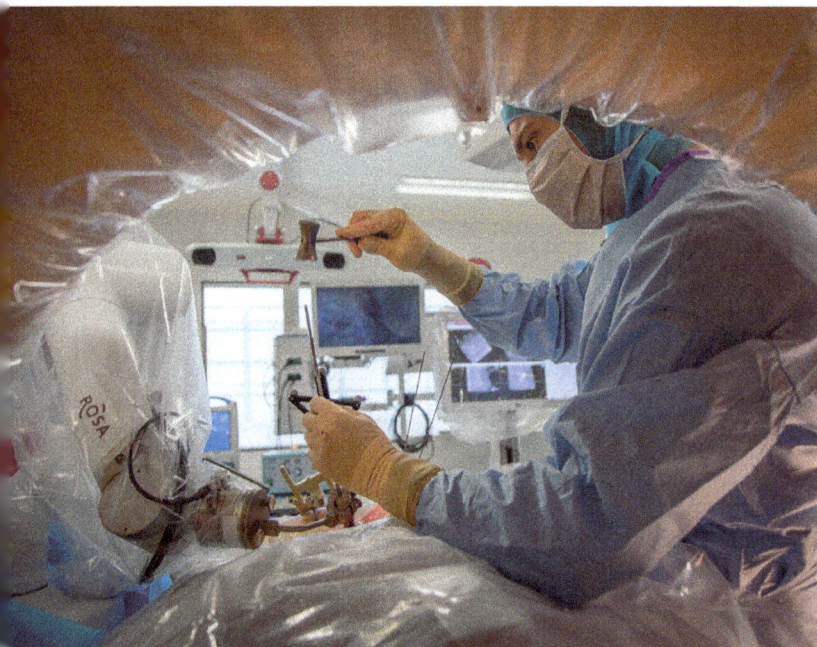

**Reducing difficulty.** Robots make complex procedures simpler and less stressful. During spinal surgery, a robot can keep the instruments perfectly still and in the correct alignment as the human surgeon drills into the bone. Traditionally, surgeons had to perform these two tasks simultaneously. This is mentally taxing and possibly dangerous since the surgeon must drill near delicate nerves. With robotic assistants, surgeons focus on their careful work. Operations are performed faster, and patients are under anesthetic for less time. Surgical robots continue to advance. The Ottava surgical robot will feature six arms to provide more control and flexibility.

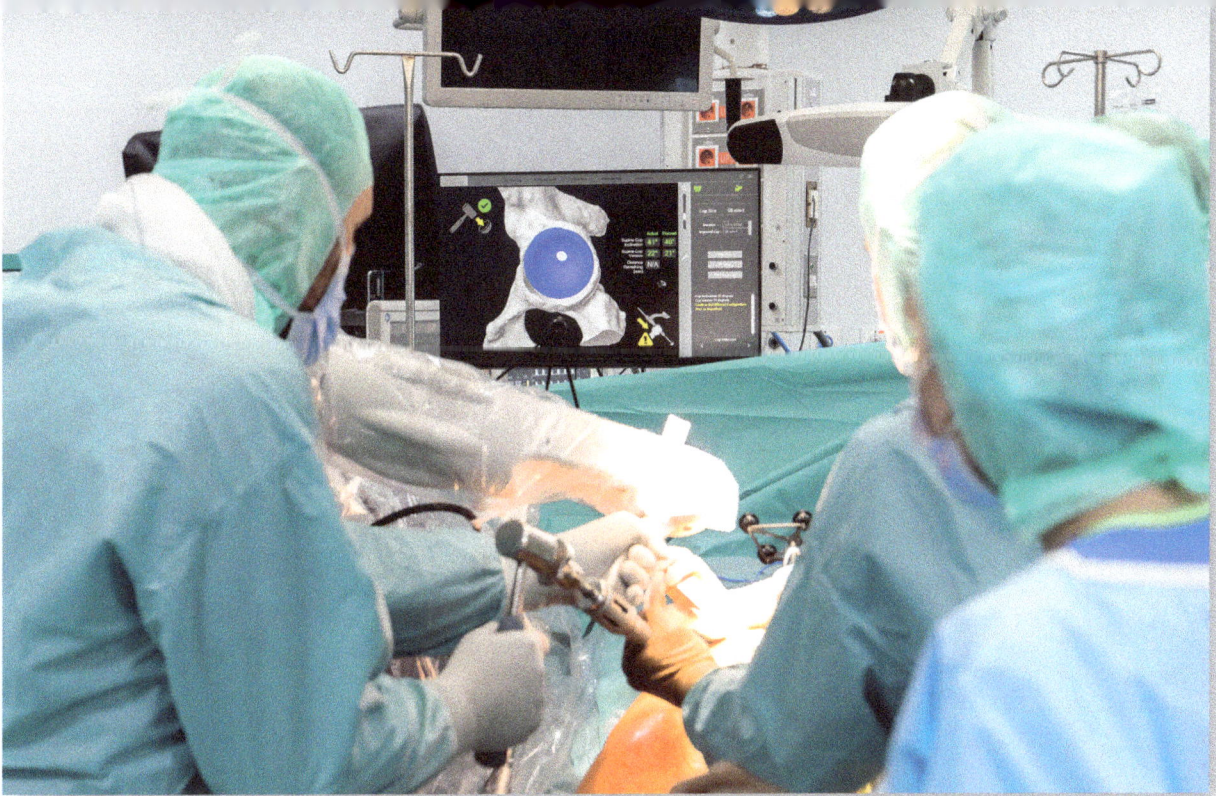

**Orthopedic surgery.** Many orthopedic procedures, such as hip and knee replacements, are performed with the help of robots. The robots combine highly maneuverable robotic arms, AI, and machine vision. With AI, robots can be trained in particular types of orthopedic surgery, learn from previous experience, and even assist surgeons in decision-making. Machine vision enables robots to differentiate between different types of tissue, so surgeons can avoid harming nerves and muscles. The Senhance surgical robot, launched in 2021, can recognize certain objects, enhance images, and carry out 3D measurements in real time.

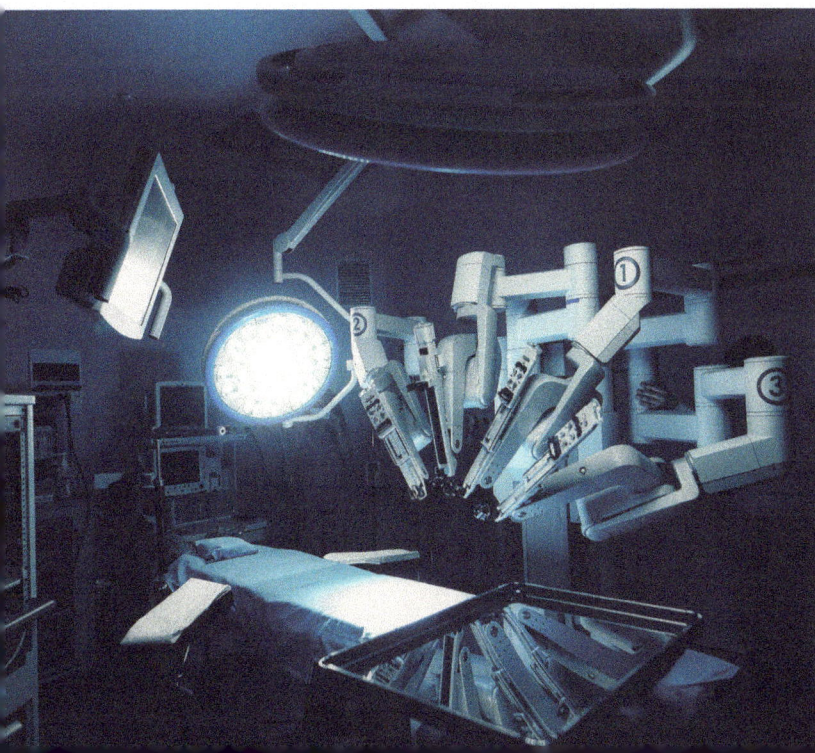

**Autonomous robotic surgery.** In 2022, a robot named STAR (Smart Tissue Autonomous Robot) achieved a world first: performing surgery without human supervision. The operation was a complete success. The patient, however, was a pig. Will robots eventually operate **autonomously** on humans? Robots will soon perform small, clearly defined procedures—under the watchful eye of a human surgeon. One problem with autonomous robot surgeons is that if the robot makes an error and causes harm during an operation, it isn't clear who is to blame.

# AUTONOMOUS MOBILE ROBOTS

Autonomous mobile robots (AMR's) are hospital workhorses, carrying out such routine tasks as delivering meals and medicines to patients, restocking medical supplies, and transporting laundry. They lower the risk of infectious disease by reducing human-to-human contact. They also help with heavy lifting, such as moving beds and patients, easing the physical strain on hospital workers.

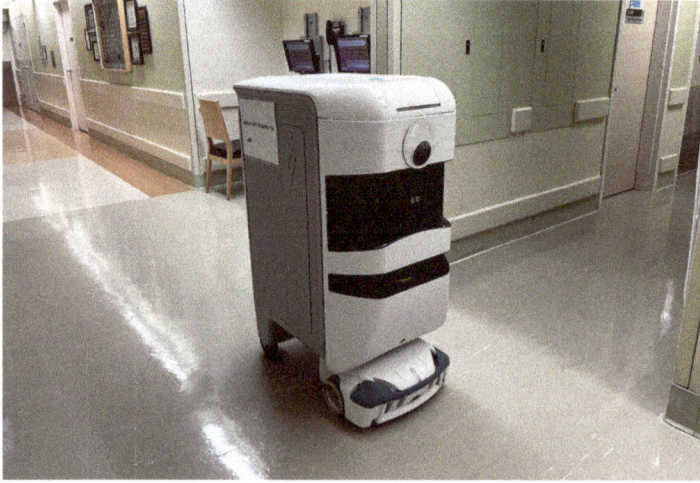

**Self-navigation.** AMR's navigate themselves around the hospital according to programmed routes. They avoid obstacles by using LiDAR (light detection and ranging). A LiDAR device emits repeated pulses of light. The light bounces back to a sensor after striking an object, and the robot steers around it. Such AMR's as Yujin Robot's GoCart can make deliveries as fast as human workers. They can be programmed to make multiple stops and can adapt to changes in routes and schedules.

**Cleaning.** Exposure to *pathogens* (germs) is always a risk in hospitals. Robots are used to clean and sanitize hospital rooms to keep human workers safe. AMR's wash and scrub floors and use high-intensity ultraviolet (UV) light—which kills germs—to disinfect rooms. UV light is dangerous to humans, so AMR's use motion sensors to detect any people in the vicinity.

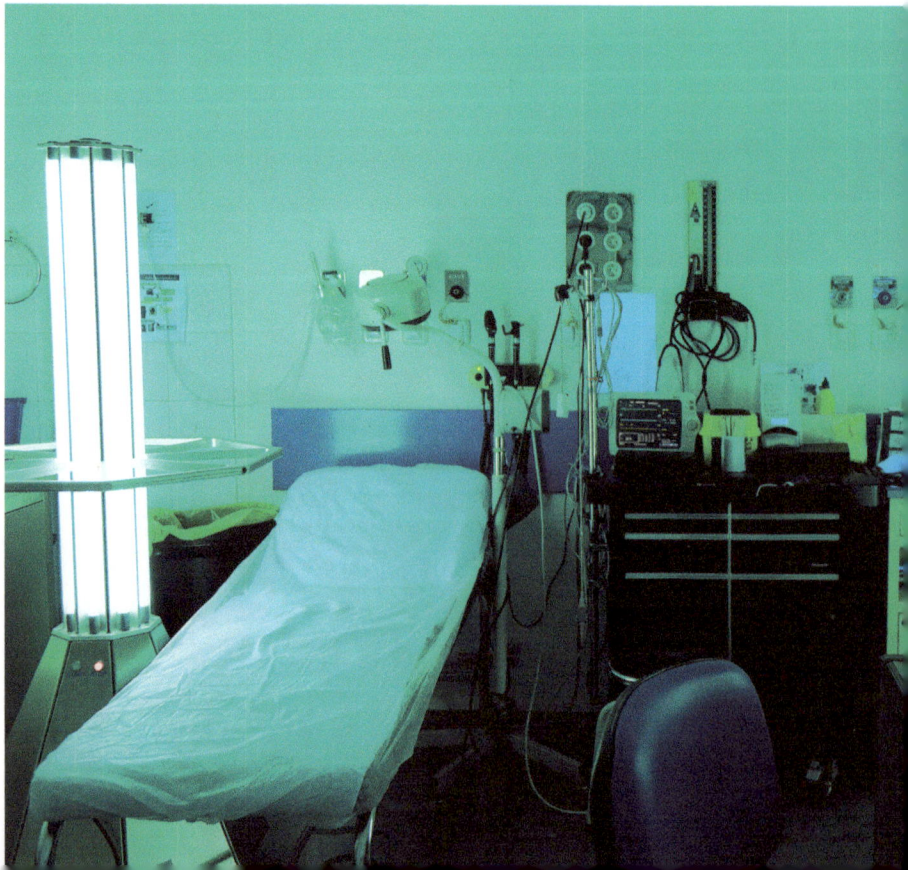

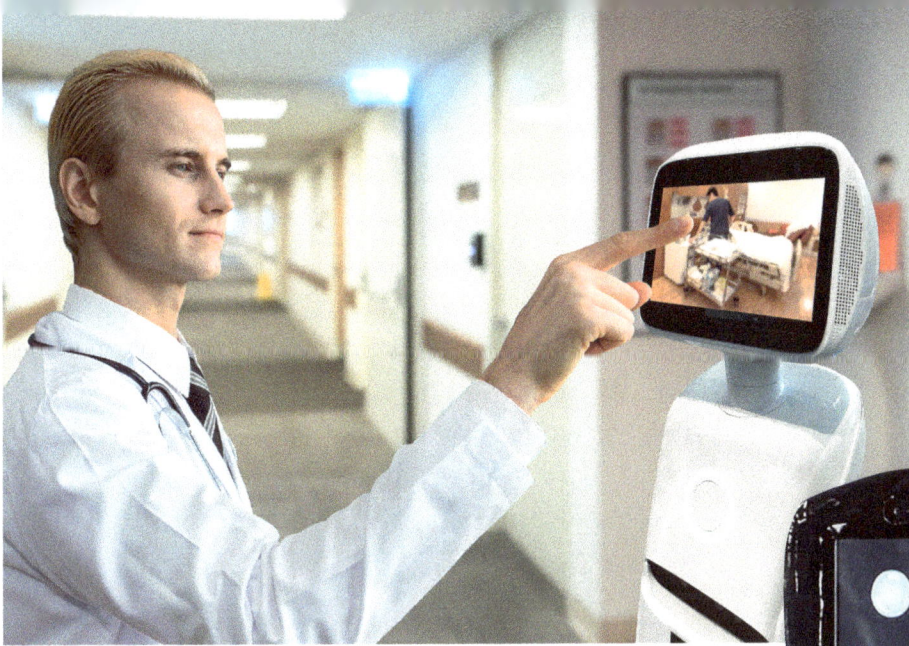

**Consultations and visits.** Sometimes a doctor cannot meet face-to-face with a patient—during a **pandemic,** for example. In such cases, AMR's provide a remote link. A doctor can consult with a patient via a computer screen on the AMR. The AMR's can also host video calls between patients and their loved ones. AMR's accompanying doctors on hospital rounds contribute advice on diagnosis or treatment.

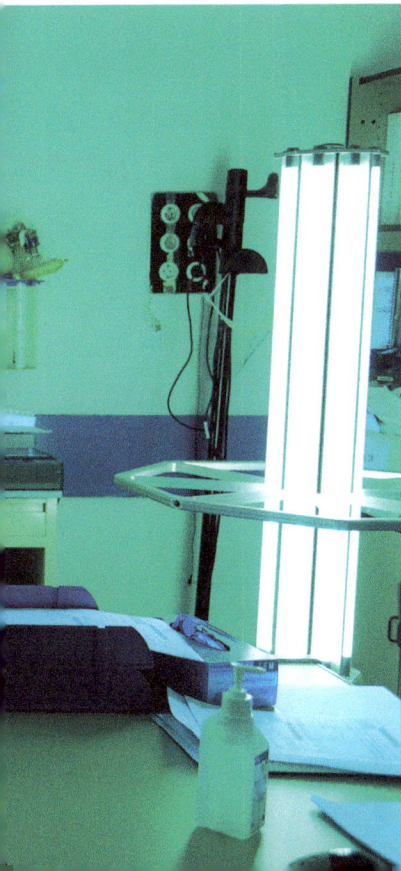

**Triage** occurs in an emergency room (ER) where patients are treated in order of priority, with the most urgent cases treated first. A hospital in Mexico uses an AMR named RoomieBot to triage patients as they arrive in the ER. RoomieBot uses AI and machine vision to take a patient's temperature, blood oxygen level, and medical history. RoomieBot's AI decides the patient's urgency and allocates the patient to a doctor.

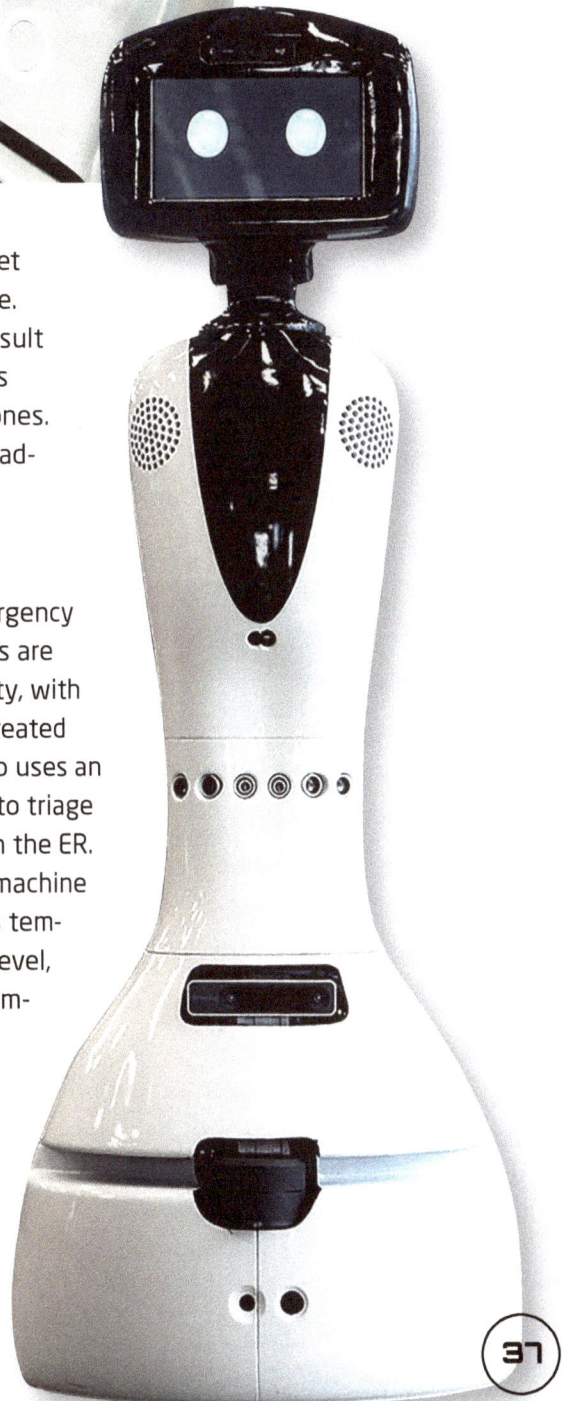

37

# CARE, SUPPORT, AND REHABILITATION

Friendliness, patience, and sensitivity are not traits we necessarily associate with machines. Yet robots increasingly play a role as carers and companions for seniors and those with long-term care needs in hospitals and at home. Robotic devices are being used to support and **rehabilitate** people with injured or paralyzed limbs.

**Robotic exoskeletons.** Robotic exoskeletons are used by people with weak or paralyzed limbs caused by a stroke or spinal injury. The exoskeletons are strapped to the user's limbs to help with standing, walking, lifting, and carrying. Exoskeletons use battery-powered motors to drive movement. As the user shifts their weight, sensors activate motors to initiate movement. A human therapist can adjust the power of the limb to suit the user. The power and degree of movement allowed are adjusted as treatment progresses.

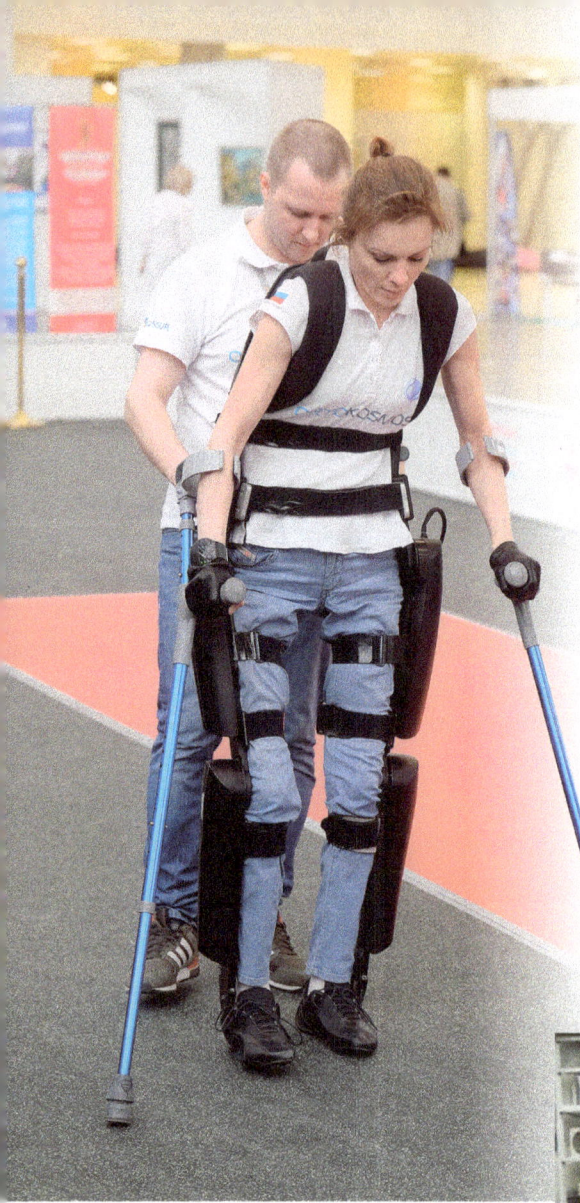

**Robotic arm.** Wheelchair-mounted robotic arms help patients with spinal injuries perform daily tasks, such as eating, drinking, and writing. The robotic arm is controlled by an AI neural network that adapts to the user's needs and provides real-time error correction as the arm manipulates objects.

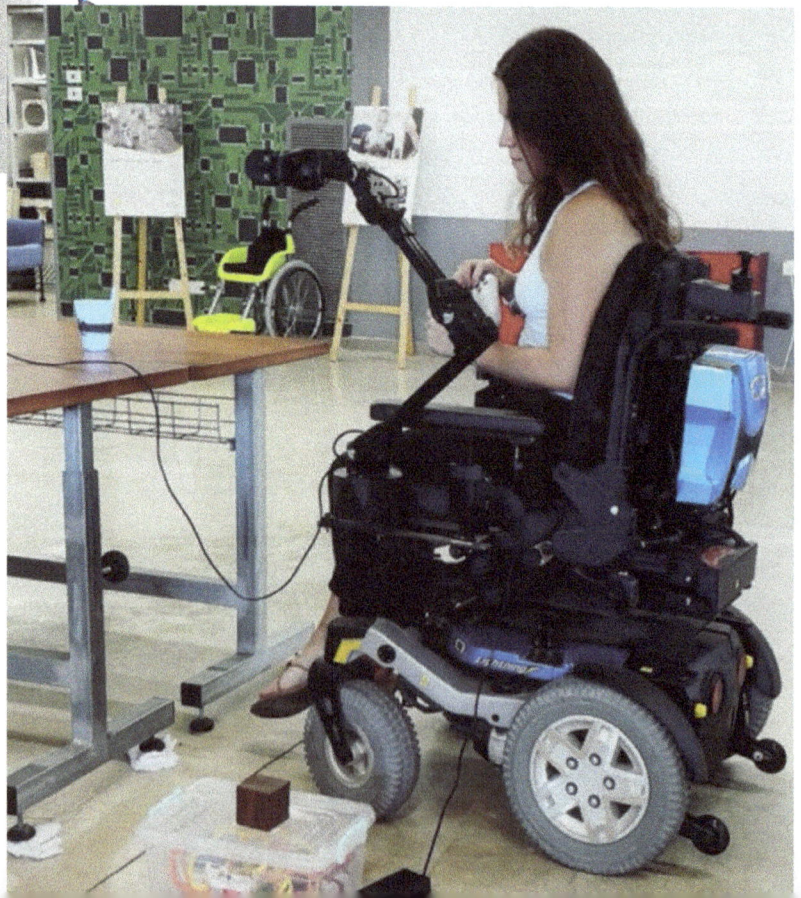

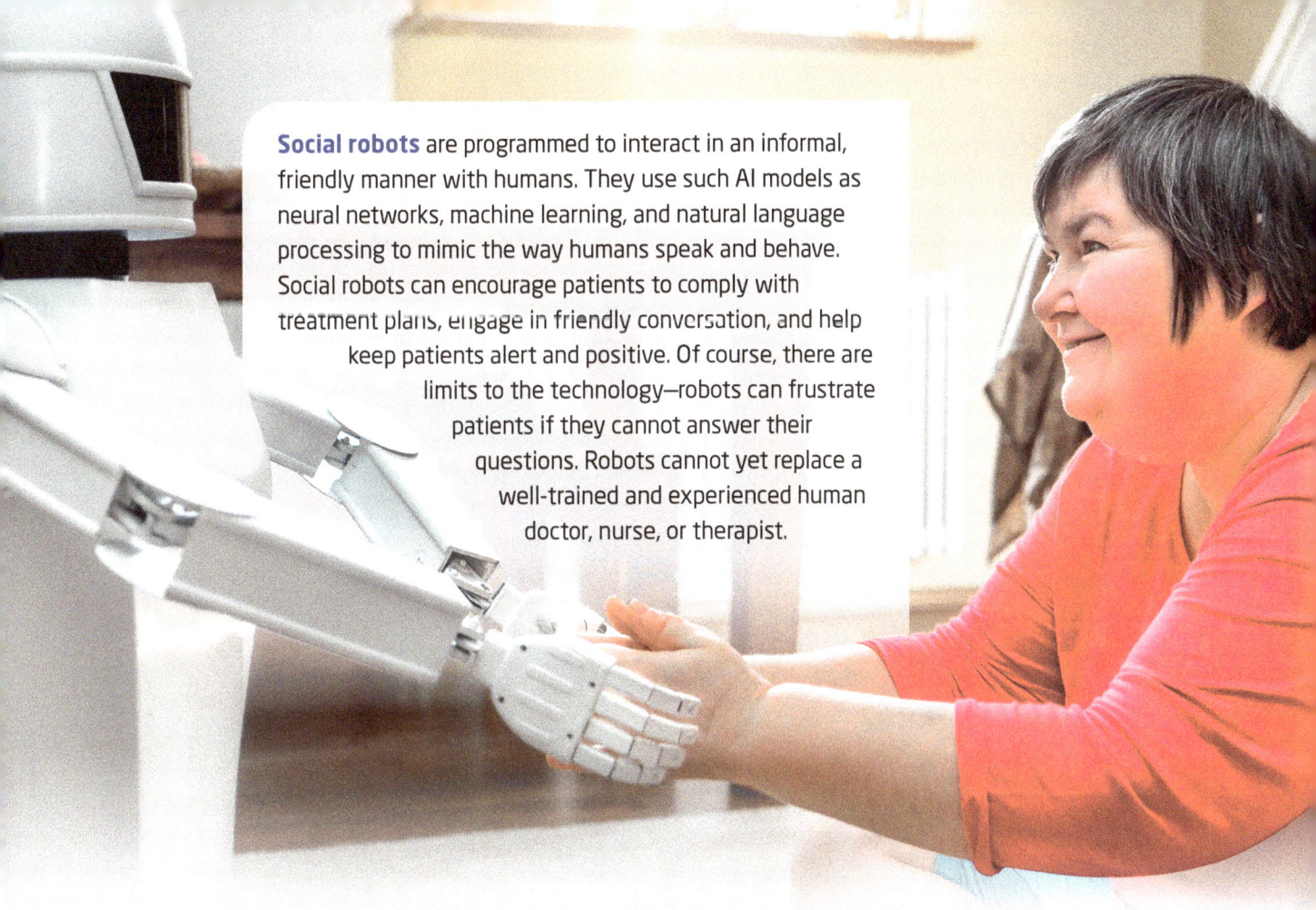

**Social robots** are programmed to interact in an informal, friendly manner with humans. They use such AI models as neural networks, machine learning, and natural language processing to mimic the way humans speak and behave. Social robots can encourage patients to comply with treatment plans, engage in friendly conversation, and help keep patients alert and positive. Of course, there are limits to the technology—robots can frustrate patients if they cannot answer their questions. Robots cannot yet replace a well-trained and experienced human doctor, nurse, or therapist.

**Robotic prosthetic limbs.** Researchers have developed robotic arms for amputees, controlled by electric signals from the user's nerves and muscles. Users use their mind to manipulate a robotic arm to feed themselves. Robotic hands can even experience a sense of touch! Scientists have built robotic legs that adjust to walking on sloping or rough terrain, climbing stairs, squatting, and running. The robotic legs are controlled by switches and sensors on the device rather than a user's mind. The risks of a connection failure are too great for a user climbing stairs. But technological challenges remain. Robotic limbs need to be lighter, less noisy, and have longer battery life.

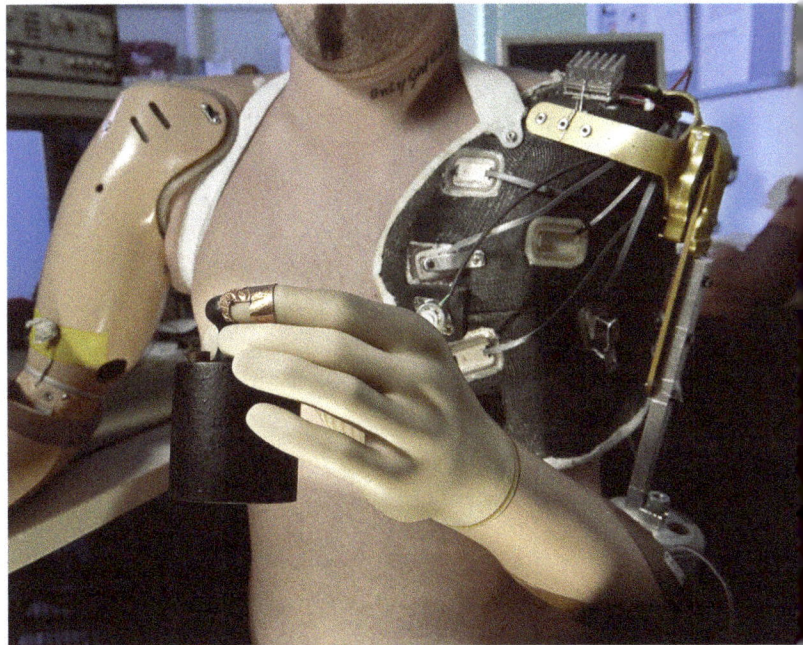

# 6 VIRTUAL REALITY

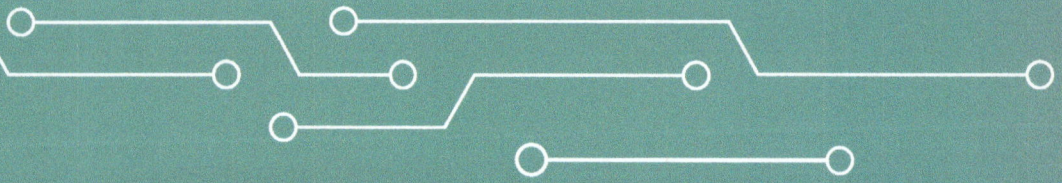

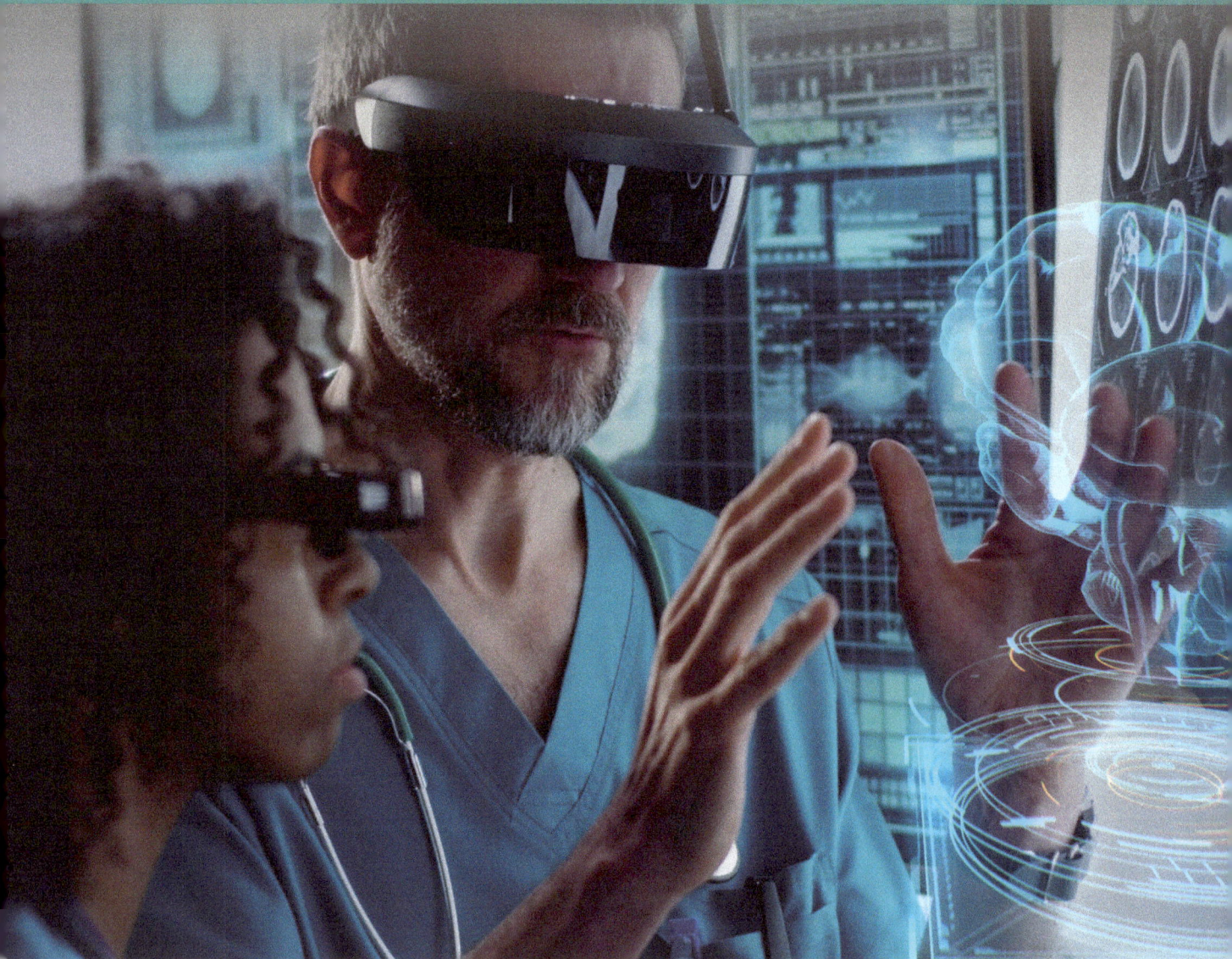

# IMMERSIVE, INTERACTIVE, AND SENSORY

You may think of virtual reality (VR) only as entertainment. But VR has important applications in health and medicine. VR is a technology where users enter an immersive, computer-generated simulation of reality. When users put on a VR headset, the outside environment vanishes—instantly replaced by a 360-degree virtual world they move around and interact with. Users wear **haptic** gloves to provide sensory feedback, so they can see, hear, and touch in this virtual world.

VR is used in medical training, allowing medical students to experience a 3D simulation of a surgical procedure. VR is a useful device for doctors when explaining a medical condition or treatment to anxious patients and their families. VR is also effective for pain management and therapy for people suffering from anxiety, depression, and addiction. VR may not work for everyone or in every situation, but it is fast becoming an established tool for medical education, surgery, pain control, and therapy.

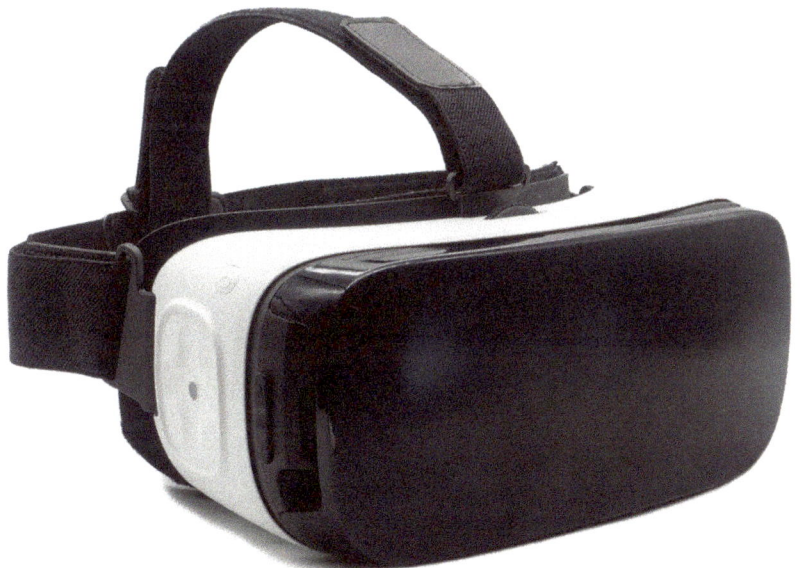

# SURGERY

Surgery is complex and stressful, requiring split-second decision-making where the wrong choice can lead to serious harm or death. VR can help train surgeons, assist in presurgery planning, and is even used in operations. VR's immersive, interactive, and sensory nature makes it an ideal environment for doctors to learn the skills they need.

**Virtual anatomy.** Medical students use VR to examine the body's physical structures at close range. They can virtually miniaturize themselves and venture inside a beating heart and watch the blood flow within its chambers. This form of learning goes beyond the capabilities of any medical textbook. VR dissection may eventually replace human *cadavers* (corpses) for medical students studying human anatomy.

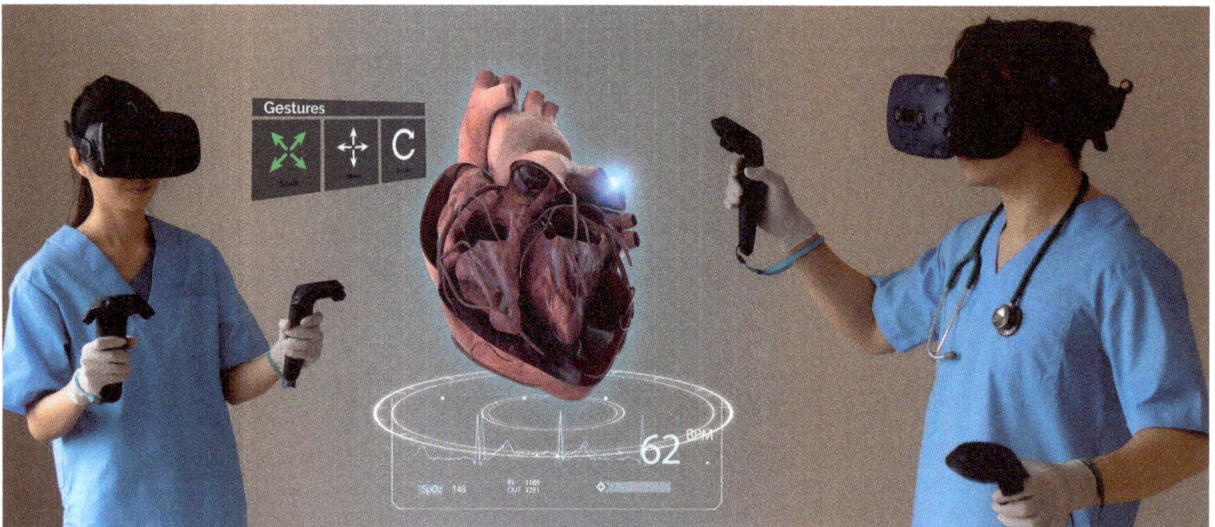

**Surgical training.** Medical students can now don VR goggles to enter a virtual operating room and practice surgery on a virtual patient. Haptic technology enables students to feel virtual instruments, cut into virtual flesh, and suture virtual incisions. VR simulations use imagery from real-life operations filmed in high definition from every angle. But VR is no replacement for a real human cadaver, and it cannot fully reproduce the sensation of handling surgical instruments in a real body. Some patients may not feel comfortable with a surgeon trained only in VR.

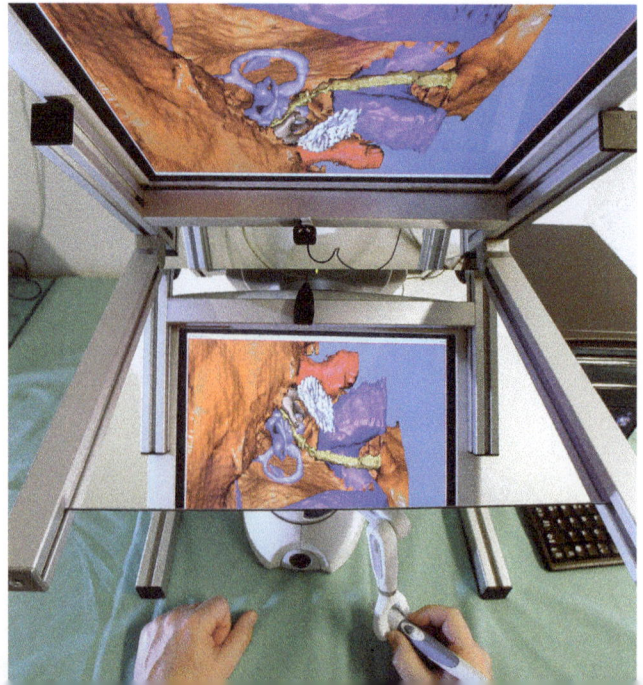

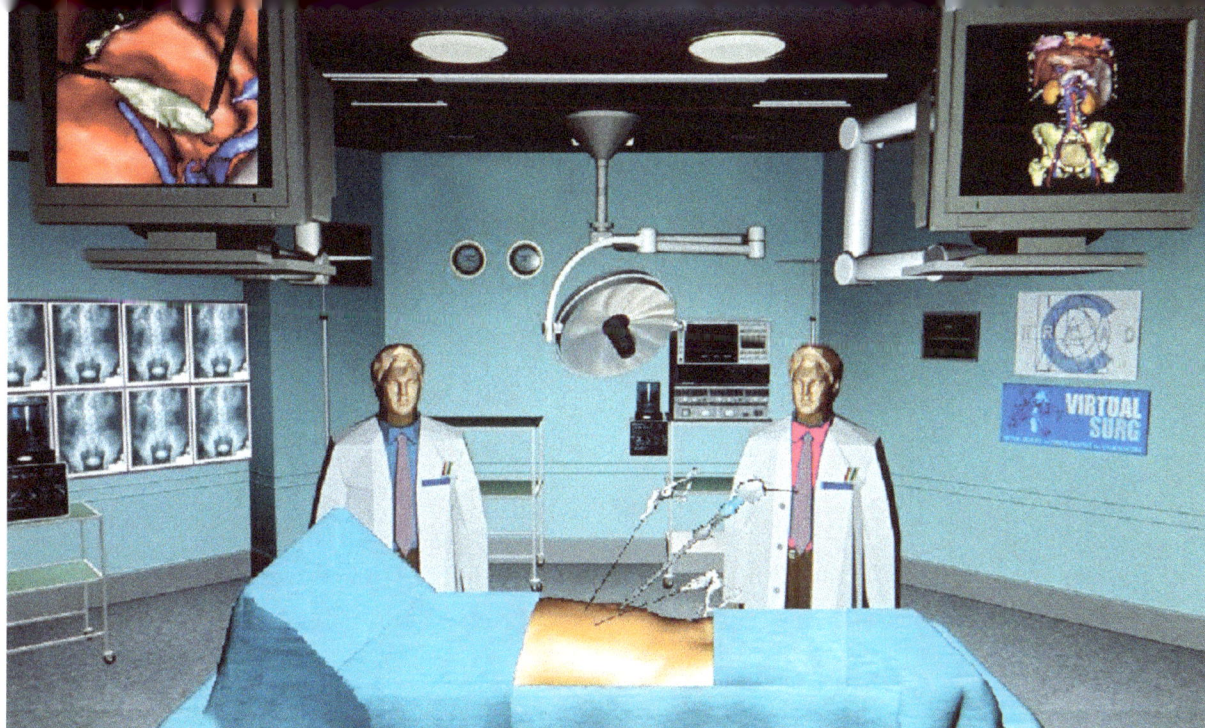

**Planning surgery.** VR is used to plan complex surgical procedures. VR surgical plans use a magnified 3D simulation of the surgical site compiled from MRI scans and other medical imagery. The surgical team, linked by VR headsets, can walk through the surgery and discuss the best approach. A company named ImmersiveTouch equips surgeons with virtual tools to physically rehearse a surgical procedure. Planning and rehearsing an operation means patients spend less time in the operating room under anesthesia.

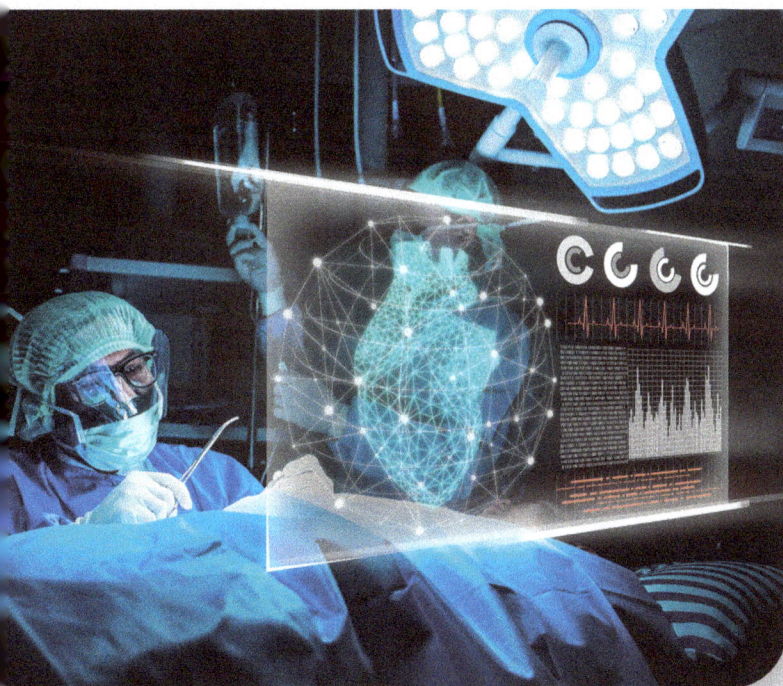

**VR robotic surgery.** In robotic surgery, a robotic arm is controlled by a human surgeon at a **console.** The surgeon receives images of the operation site from a camera positioned within the body. VR gives a surgeon more direct experience—providing tactile and sensory feedback as they maneuver instruments from the console. A VR company named Augmedics offers surgeons "X-ray vision capabilities," allowing them to see through obstructions as they operate. SentiAR provides real-time VR information on patient health throughout the surgery. SentiAR uses augmented reality (AR) technology, where a surgeon can reference images that appear to float above a patient.

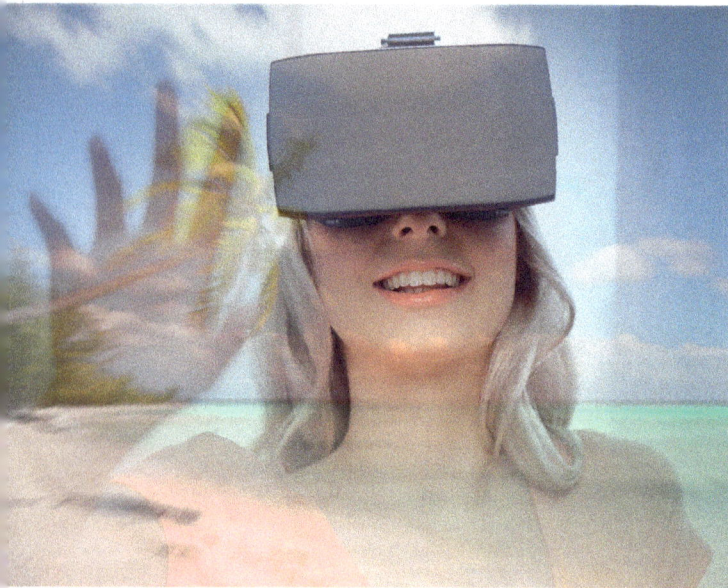

# THERAPY, PAIN MANAGEMENT, AND REHABILITATION

You are lying on a tropical beach. Above you is a bright blue sky. The sand is white, palm trees move gently in the breeze, and you hear distant waves on the shore. The experience feels real, but it's not. In fact, you are lying in a hospital bed having suffered a serious injury. But all that seems far away inside this virtual world. Even the pain seems much less severe.

**Pain management.** Virtual reality feels real, and that is why it is effective at reducing pain and suffering. Your brain cannot live in two realities at once. So it accepts the given VR input. If you see yourself on a beautiful VR beach, it's harder to focus on other sensations and pain. Researchers find that VR therapy can reduce pain for people suffering from burns, lower back pain, stomach pain, arthritis, and cancer. It even reduces the pain of childbirth. VR pain management reduces the need for pain-relieving drugs. Mental health workers trained in VR therapy are called virtualists. They help patients decide on the best virtual experience and advise them on the use of VR in their therapy.

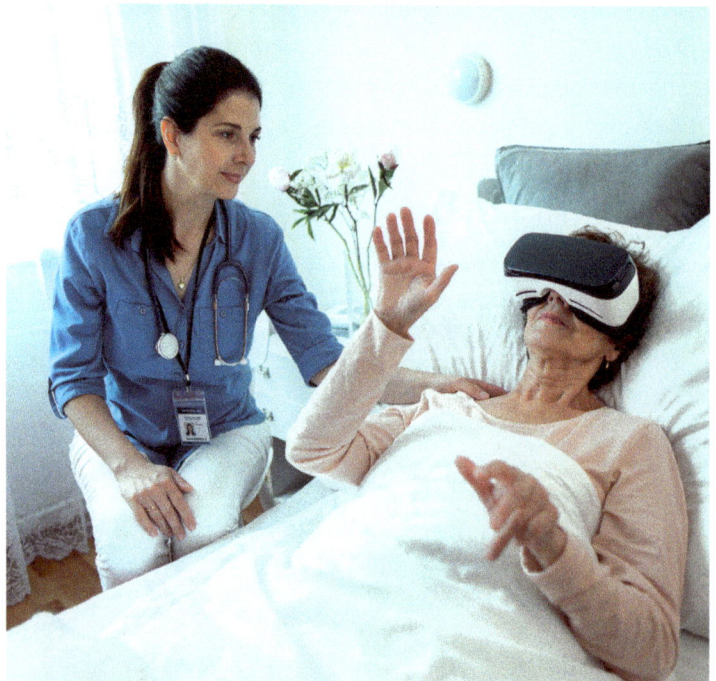

**Medical procedure anxiety.** Cancer patients undergoing *chemotherapy* (drug treatment) often suffer from stress, anxiety, discomfort, and boredom. Some hospitals now offer VR headsets, so cancer patients can virtually transport themselves from their dull surroundings to a mountain lake, a flower-filled meadow, or a coral reef. VR games help distract anxious children who fear injections and other medical treatments.

**Physical therapy and rehabilitation.** Therapists use VR to help people recover from strokes and injuries. The immersive VR experience helps motivate patients to do more than they think they can. Absorbed in a VR world, patients are distracted from their pain—making it easier to exercise. This way, VR helps shorten rehabilitation and recovery time.

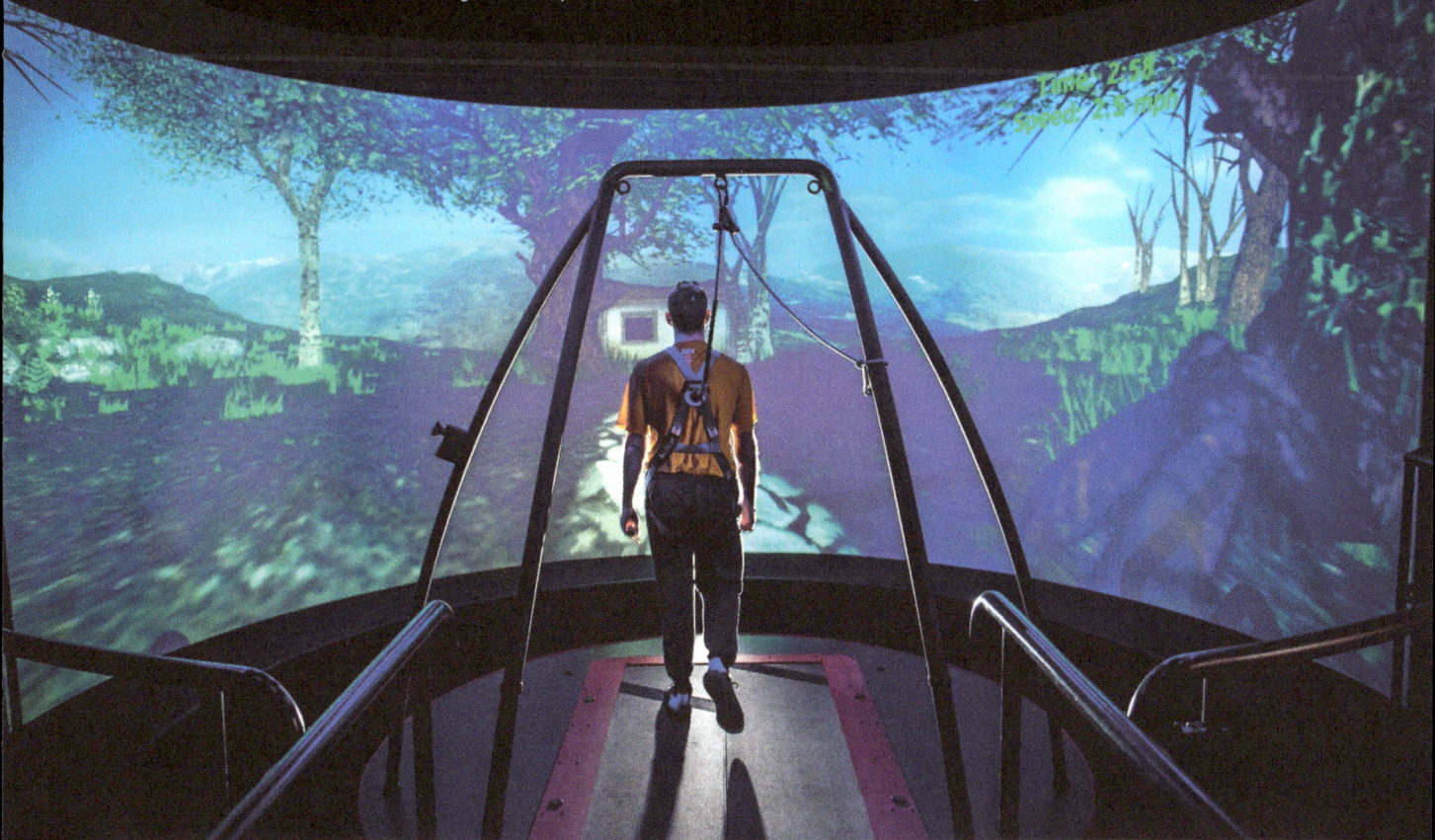

**Mental health.** Patients who struggle to face their fears in real life may be able to do so in virtual reality. VR is used to treat patients with *agoraphobia* (fear of open or crowded places), *acrophobia* (fear of heights), and post-traumatic stress disorder (PTSD), a condition triggered by a traumatic experience. Through VR, patients increase their exposure to fear triggers gradually under therapist supervision. VR also helps treat people recovering from drug or alcohol addiction. Patients virtually expose themselves to addiction urges in a simulated VR setting to practice resisting the urges.

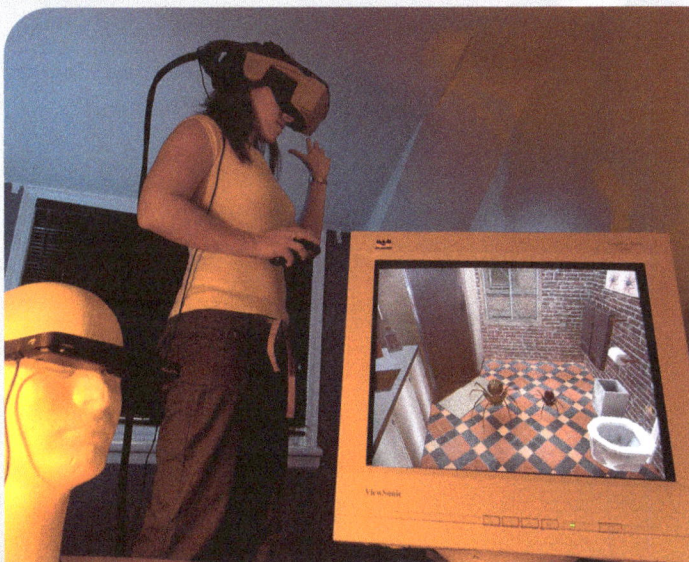

# ENGAGE YOUR READER

Nonfiction writing often includes subject-specific vocabulary terms. Knowing the words related to the topic helps us understand the text itself.

When good readers come upon words they don't know well, they pause and try to figure them out. One tool they use is the glossary, like the one on page 4. Not every word can be defined in a glossary, though!

Authors know this, so they leave clues about words in the text. Next time you encounter a challenging word, stop and look for information about its meaning in the surrounding sentences. Sometimes authors define the term right there in the text! Other times, they'll compare the term to something you may already know. Authors even use punctuation like commas or dashes to clue you in to a word's meaning.

## INSTRUCTIONS

1. Consider the list of challenge words and identify where each is used in the text. You can use the Index on page 48 to help you locate each term.

2. Explain how the author described each word. Ask yourself "what is happening in the text?" or "how is this word being used?" as you search for clues about their meanings.

3. Create your own definitions of the words. Don't just copy the dictionary definitions. Instead think about how you would tell a friend what each term means.

4. Add a visual representation for each word. Think about what you could draw that will help you remember what the words mean.

## CHALLENGE WORDS

- Synthetic organs
- Compatibility
- Stem cells
- Wearables

- Nanoparticles
- Biomarkers
- Autonomous
- Virtual reality (VR)

# EXAMPLE

| Challenge Word | Page(s) | Author's Description | Personal Definition | Visual Representation |
|---|---|---|---|---|
| Synthetic organs | 7-11 | - something synthetic is something artificial<br>- synthetic organs have been custom-created in laboratories | An artificial organ that can be used to replace unhealthy organs in sick individuals. They are made from the patient's own cells along with stem cells or bioprinting. Synthetic organs have lower rejection rates. | |
| Compatibility | | | | |

# INDEX

www.ingramcontent.com/pod-product-compliance
Lightning Source LLC
Chambersburg PA
CBHW040144200326
41519CB00032B/7593